# Praise for *Soccer Injury Preve*

"The health and welfare of our players is a top priority. As a major league sport, we are constantly evaluating our programs and procedures to ensure our athletes are operating at peak performance. In *Soccer Injury Prevention and Treatment*, John Gallucci has done a terrific job outlining some of the most common soccer injuries and explaining what any athletes can do—from an amateur to a professional—to prevent injuries before they occur. John's book serves as an important resource for soccer players of all ages and abilities."

—Don Garber, Commissioner of Major League Soccer

"During my more than 30 years working in soccer in the United States, the game has developed in many areas on and off the field. While not always discussed, injury prevention is an important aspect in helping us continue to grow the game at all levels. *Soccer Injury Prevention and Treatment* does an outstanding job at delivering expert advice on injuries and how to prevent them. John Gallucci Jr.'s insight provides parents, coaches, and players with an invaluable soccer medicine resource."

—Sunil Gulati, President, United States Soccer Federation

"As a player who experienced a handful of nagging injuries throughout my career, I know firsthand how important it is to take the time to prepare your body for the rigors of your sport. This book not only describes common soccer injuries and the treatment process, but goes into detail about how to prevent these injuries to keep you on the field and at 100%. The knowledge and resources outlined in John Gallucci's book would have been invaluable to me if available during my tenure as a professional athlete."

—Claudio Reyna, Sporting Director, New York FC

"I have had a lifelong interest in sports medicine, stretching back to my days as a high school and college athlete. Throughout my career I have served as head orthopedic surgeon for a handful of professional sports teams, including the New York Red Bulls. During my experiences, I have seen countless injuries and have always stressed the importance of education to not only my patients, but their coaches and parents as well. John's book does a great job of giving a true understanding of sports medicine knowledge, written and executed in a way that makes it easy to follow, understand, and absorb."

—Dr. Decter, Former New York Red Bulls Team Physician

"I've known John for the past 10 years and can attest to his dedication and commitment to his patients and practice. John was instrumental in keeping me in peak shape to perform at an elite level even into my late thirties. This book is a must read for any athlete who plays sports. The lessons and practices in this book are invaluable and can help you perform at your best!"

—Jeff Agoos, Vice President of Competition, Major League Soccer

"An excellent book! I've worked closely for many years with John Gallucci to offer the highest quality sports medicine care and resources for the athletes of Major League Soccer. In 2001, I founded the National Center for Sports Safety after identifying a need to decrease the number and severity of injuries to youth, recreational, and high school athletes. *Soccer Injury Prevention and Treatment* follows the same principles and gives the reader a wealth of information about common soccer injuries, and more importantly, proactive preventive measures."

—Dr. Larry Lemak, Medical Director of Major League Soccer

"I've been treating and researching sports specific musculoskeletal injuries for nearly two decades and I'm confident in saying that *Soccer Injury Prevention and Treatment* is an exceptional tool for medical professionals and athletes alike. This book covers it all, from nutrition to concussions and injuries of all kinds. It's second to none for knowledge on prevention and getting players back out on the pitch after injury."

—Dr. John G. Kennedy, Orthopedic Surgeon, Hospital for
Special Surgery, New York, NY

"I'd like to say I've seen it all when it comes to injuries, both during my years as a professional soccer player and now as a youth coach. You always hate to see a player on the sidelines due to injury, and as a coach I am constantly educating my athletes on how to properly prepare for the game of soccer. John does a great job of using his expertise and knowledge and putting it out there for the masses to utilize. As a former athlete and coach, and as a parent, this book is a must read!"

—Tony Meola, U.S. Soccer Hall of Fame Goalkeeper

"*Soccer Injury Prevention and Treatment* is a great resource for athletes looking to compete and progress on the soccer field. The attention to detail that John utilizes while describing each injury makes it relatable to parents, players, and coaches as they educate themselves on common soccer injuries. As a sports medicine physician, I am always preaching that "prevention is key," and this book thoroughly outlines techniques used to prevent injuries, not only in text form, but by providing pictures and charts that make the content relatable and easy to understand."

—Dr. Hutter, Former Assistant New York Red Bulls Team Physician

"As Senior Director of Supporter Relations and Safety at Major League Soccer, I too often see players out due to injury. *Soccer Injury Prevention and Treatment* is a great go-to guide for the non-medical professional, explaining what you need to know in detail, defining terms, and providing visuals to supplement the text. John Gallucci helps players, coaches, and parents by providing education and understanding about the causes of injuries and the proper path to recovery."

—Evan Dabby, Senior Director of Supporter Relations and Safety, Major League Soccer

"Soccer has been in my life since the day I was born. My father is a long-time coach, and at the age of sixteen I signed my first professional contract with Major League Soccer. Throughout my youth years I sustained several injuries, and John Gallucci assisted in my care. John's *Soccer Injury Prevention and Treatment* does a great job of taking the questions that players, coaches, and parents have regarding soccer injuries, and thoroughly explains the entire process from start to finish. More important, the emphasis on injury prevention serves as a great resource for athletes at all levels, because no matter what level you play at, the last thing you want to do is watch from the sidelines."

—Michael Bradley, Professional Soccer Player, Toronto FC, U.S. National Team

"I have sent numerous patients to John over my many years in practice and they have had not only exceptional care but have been able to return to high level of sport. He has also instructed many of my non-surgical patients in prevention programs, which has had much success in helping to prevent lower extremity injuries. *Soccer Injury Prevention and Treatment* is a must-read for parents, players, and coaches throughout the soccer community."

—Dr. Beth Shubin Stein, Orthopedic Surgeon, Hospital for Special Surgery

"Having worked as a team physician throughout all levels of athletics, I put a huge emphasis on keeping my athletes physically fit and at the top of their game. Unfortunately, injuries do happen, and when they do it is my job to get that athlete back to 100% as quickly and effectively as possible. In *Soccer Injury Prevention and Treatment*, John Gallucci Jr. does a great job of providing education on the recovery process, allowing parents, players, and coaches to take a proactive approach in getting back on the soccer field."

—Dr. Riley J. Williams, Orthopedic Surgeon, Hospital for Special Surgery, Head Team Physician, New York Red Bulls

"John Gallucci was an integral part of my success as a soccer player at Harvard University. John understands what it takes physically, mentally, and emotionally to compete at the highest level. Not only does John provide exceptional treatment, he is a specialist in injury prevention, focusing on individualized care well beyond return to sport. Thanks to John I was able to be the best and healthiest athlete that I could be."

—Katherine Sheeleigh, 2010 Ivy League Player of the Year, Soccer America All-American

# SOCCER INJURY PREVENTION AND TREATMENT

# SOCCER INJURY PREVENTION AND TREATMENT

## A Guide to Optimal Performance for Players, Parents, and Coaches

John Gallucci, Jr., MS, ATC, PT, DPT

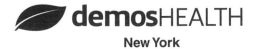

**New York**

**Visit our website at www.demoshealth.com**

*ISBN:* 978-1-936303-65-6
*e-book ISBN:* 978-1-61705-219-4

*Acquisitions Editor:* Julia Pastore
*Compositor:* diacriTech

Medical information provided by Demos Health, in the absence of a visit with a health care professional, must be considered as an educational service only. This book is not designed to replace a physician's independent judgment about the appropriateness or risks of a procedure or therapy for a given patient. Our purpose is to provide you with information that will help you make your own health care decisions.

The information and opinions provided here are believed to be accurate and sound, based on the best judgment available to the authors, editors, and publisher, but readers who fail to consult appropriate health authorities assume the risk of injuries. The publisher is not responsible for errors or omissions. The editors and publisher welcome any reader to report to the publisher any discrepancies or inaccuracies noticed.

**Library of Congress Cataloging-in-Publication Data**

Gallucci, John.
    Soccer injury prevention and treatment : a guide to optimal performance for players, parents and coaches / John Gallucci, Jr., MS, ATC, PT, DPT.
        pages cm
    ISBN 978-1-936303-65-6 — ISBN 978167105214 (e-book)
    1. Soccer injuries—Prevention. 2. Soccer injuries—Treatment.
    I. Title.
    RC1220.S57G34 2014
    617.1'0276334—dc23
                            2014006963

Special discounts on bulk quantities of Demos Health books are available to corporations, professional associations, pharmaceutical companies, health care organizations, and other qualifying groups. For details, please contact:

Special Sales Department
Demos Medical Publishing, LLC
11 West 42nd Street, 15th Floor
New York, NY 10036
Phone: 800-532-8663 or 212-683-0072
Fax: 212-941-7842
E-mail: specialsales@demosmedical.com

Printed in the United States of America by McNaughton & Gunn Printing.
14 15 16 17 18 / 5 4 3 2 1

*I would like to dedicate this book to my wife, Dawn, and my children, Stephanie and Charlie. Your support and love help me persevere each and every day. Your smiles give me the drive to go after my dreams and accomplish my goals.*

# CONTENTS

# FOREWORD

*Tabaré (Tab) Ramos Ricciardi was born in Uruguay, and emigrated to the United States with his family in 1978. They settled in New Jersey, where Ramos was a soccer star at St. Benedict's Preparatory School in Newark. He went on to play at North Carolina State University, where he was a three-time All-American. Ramos played professionally for 13 seasons in Spain, Mexico, and the United States. He was the first player to sign with Major League Soccer, where he played seven years and was a three-time All-Star with the MetroStars. Ramos's U.S. National Team career began in 1988 and ended in 2000, and included three World Cup appearances. He was elected to the National Soccer Hall of Fame in 2005 and to the U.S. Soccer Federation 100th Anniversary All-Time Best XI in 2013. He is currently the U.S. Soccer Federation Youth Technical Director and head coach of the U.S. U-20 national team.*

I basically grew up with a soccer ball at my feet. My father played professionally in Uruguay, for CA River Plate in Montevideo, but my mother was actually the bigger fan of the game. I always remember her in the kitchen, cooking something with a soccer game on in the background. There wasn't a lot of soccer on TV back then, so she'd find a tape of an old game or watch a replay of a game on Univision. My mom and I really connected because she watched soccer all the time.

And I played it all the time.

We came to this country when I was 11 years old. It was strange and difficult for me. I had taken English classes in Uruguay, but I could only say things like "the cat is under the table." Nothing useful. So I spent about six months playing soccer by myself on the playground, just kicking the ball around on my own. And then one day, a kid came up and asked to play with me, and asked if I was interested in signing up for recreational soccer. I did, and I played for one day.

The field was too small and I was way too advanced. They took me to a travel team in Kearny, which had a lot of people with European backgrounds. I began playing with the children of immigrants from Ireland and Scotland and other countries where soccer is the most popular sport. Playing sports always helps you make friends, so being involved in soccer really helped me at that time. Being a good player made it even easier to meet people, make friends, and be accepted into the culture.

There wasn't a point when I realized a pro career was going to happen, but my motivation was always to play professional soccer. It was all I wanted since I was six or seven years old. All my parents wanted was for me to get an education, so for them, that was what mattered. Today, games are so important to players and to parents, but to my parents, how I did in school was what was really important. A bad grade in school meant I was not allowed to play soccer, end of story. It didn't matter if it was a regional final or just another indoor game. My coaches would call, and my parents would just say, he's not playing, that's it.

Things are so different now. Parents are so involved. Probably too involved. My father would be the first to say he was not very involved in my development as a soccer player. He played professionally, yes, and he would go to my games and yell, but he was not one to be involved in terms of making sure he took me to practice, or got me on the best team. There was none of that, because my parents had to go to work. If I said I had practice on Thursday at 5:00, they would tell me to find my own way if I wanted to go. So I'd find a ride or get on my bike. It's just how sports were back then, at least in my family. All the time,

I think about how much things have changed since then. I'm the broken-record parent, telling my son and my daughters over and over that they can't go anywhere by themselves. I pick them up and take them everywhere, and do my best to get them in the right situation and make sure they develop properly.

Because education was so important to my parents, there was never any question that I would go to college. University of Virginia and North Carolina State University were my final two choices, but my parents basically decided I would go to NC State because the coach was an Argentine and they could speak with him about my grades and about soccer. They didn't really want me to go far away for school, but since Uruguayans and Argentinians are basically the same people, they felt very comfortable with me going there. I remember picking up the phone one day and hearing the NC State coach saying, "Congratulations, welcome aboard!" I hadn't even decided yet, but that's where I was going. My parents had decided for me.

I made the U.S. U-20 team when I was 15 years old, and played my first game for the senior national team when I was 21 years old. I'm happy to have played on the national team for so long, and proud to have played in the Olympic Games and the World Cup. They're all great memories. I'm also proud of being inducted into the Hall of Fame and even more importantly to be on U.S. Soccer's All-Time Best XI. All my life, I dreamed of being a professional player, but being named to the best team of all time is beyond anything I could have imagined.

I was a good player, but I also had many injuries. I didn't have anything chronic as a kid, but I had ankle issues and would miss a week here and there. We played on bad fields all the time. But I was lucky to not have anything very serious until my mid-20s. I had my first knee surgery when I was 26 years old, to repair cartilage, and I've had nine knee surgeries in total.

I played seven seasons with the MetroStars of MLS, and that's where I met John Gallucci, who was the team athletic trainer and physical therapist at the time. John was instrumental in helping me through countless soft tissue injuries; muscle strain and tendinitis plague every soccer player, but with proper care and treatment, their effects can be minimized. John's wisdom and education and his special way of handling athletes always got me back on the field.

John is still helping me today. As a coach with the Youth National Team, I'm very involved in my practices and often suffer bumps and bruises. I recently had another knee surgery, and did my rehab with John at JAG Physical Therapy. My local soccer club, the New Jersey Soccer Academy, uses John and JAG PT as athletic training and physical therapy resources for all its athletes. John's expertise is a valuable tool, and any time I have a question about the training or treatment of one of my athletes, or about myself, I find myself reaching for the phone to call him.

I know now that with some of the simple techniques available today, a lot of injuries can be prevented. Nowadays, there are so many ways to prepare that we didn't know about when I was playing. For example, I use the foam roller every day now, and I can't believe someone didn't discover that thing 20 years ago. It's such a simple concept. We don't let the U-20 kids leave without foam-rolling. I would have limited a lot of the muscle tears that I had if I had a better understanding of how to take care of my body when I played.

There are so many ways to strengthen the legs to prevent injury. At every level, injury prevention is extremely important and taken very seriously among all pro teams, and we need for that level of preparedness and awareness of how to prevent injuries to trickle down to the lower levels. Younger players and their parents and coaches need to be educated on how to specifically prepare for the sport of soccer.

For soccer, athletes need to work on speed, agility, and balance. These are all things we didn't work on in the past that are so effective for preventing injuries, and many are so easy they can be done in five minutes in your living room. It's just about spending a little extra time and being focused and dedicated to your sport.

This book is going to be a great tool for parents, coaches, and youth athletes to use to educate themselves about injuries that can happen to every soccer player and how to prevent them, and take care of them should they occur. There is so much information available now over the Internet, and a lot of it doesn't offer proper guidance and doesn't come from medical professionals. This book can help everyone wade through the sea of information and just get to what's right.

If soccer players are suffering constant injuries, they're probably not doing the right things to prepare to play. Hopefully, parents, coaches, and players will read this book and come to the soccer field better prepared. I hate to see players get discouraged due to nagging injuries and walk away from the game, because soccer is such a great sport. The running, jumping, flexing, and turning involved in soccer are all movements that bodies of all ages can really benefit from.

And soccer is fun. Of course, that counts, too.

Tab Ramos

# INTRODUCTION

As I write this book, I look back at the tremendous growth of the game of soccer over the last 25 years. According to FIFA (Fédération Internationale de Football Association, the international governing body of soccer), there are 265 million male and female players, along with five million referees and officials, actively involved in the game of soccer worldwide. That's 4% of the world's population.

Also according to FIFA, there were over 24 million Americans playing soccer as of 2006, and 30% of American households contain at least one person who plays soccer. Those figures are second only to baseball, which has always been America's game. But as Latin American immigration into the United States has increased, so has the popularity of soccer. The globalization of the game, the ongoing presence of U.S. teams in international competitions, and the continued building of soccer-specific stadiums in this country have also contributed to the popularity of the game.

A 2012 ESPN sports poll ranked soccer as the second most popular sport in the country for 12- to 24-year-olds. Soccer has also grown in popularity as a spectator sport; increasing numbers of Americans, having played the game in their youth, are now avid fans of the game.

With the rise in popularity of the sport has come an increase in the incidence of injury for soccer players of all ages. As medical coordinator for Major League Soccer (MLS) and owner of JAG Physical Therapy, I see the injury statistics first-hand; not just from MLS but also from youth leagues, international professional leagues, and the NCAA. My job responsibilities also include overseeing the medical care throughout MLS and assisting and implementing the development of our *Medical Policy and Procedures Manual*. The goal is to prevent and treat soccer injuries efficiently through top medical care and resources.

Over three million youth players are registered with U.S. Soccer, but countless players, from 6 to 75 years old, take to the field every day in the United States. This accounts for innumerable emergency room and doctor visits, along with hours and hours of rehabilitation with a physical therapy or athletic training professional similar to myself.

In February 2010, the *Journal of Pediatrics* reported that soccer has a higher injury rate than any other contact sport, such as basketball, football, field hockey, and lacrosse, with players 15 years of age and younger at a higher relative injury risk when compared with older players.

The goal in writing this book is to combine my education as an athletic trainer and physical therapist, my years of experience, and my clinical aptitude to try and keep players on the field, be they U.S. National Team players, professional players, college players, high school players, club players, or just recreational players trying to keep fit. I will give a detailed look at every joint and the common soccer injuries that affect them, and will simplify the diagnosis, mechanism, treatment, and prevention of each of these injuries. I hope this book becomes a resource for players, coaches, referees, and parents to assist in keeping our players safe, healthy, and on the pitch.

You will see many references within this book to JAG Physical Therapy's Lower Extremity Strengthening System, or LESS Program. Many lower body injuries can be prevented if the muscles of the lower body and core are strengthened in preparation for activity. The LESS Program is listed in its entirety on page 171–184 for easy incorporation into any athlete's training program.

While I was finishing my master's degree in athletic training and my doctorate in physical therapy, I was always interested in teaching athletes about how to take care of their bodies. I have always told parents, coaches, athletes, and medical professionals, "Your body is your tool. You need to take care of your tools to accomplish your goals."

Over my 22-year career, I have seen many different types of sports medicine injuries. My time with New York University, Columbia University, and the New York Knicks gave me a platform of experiences and education to prepare me for the last 16 years of my career as a sports medicine professional.

My career with MLS began when I started doing rehabilitation on surgical cases with the MetroStars. I had the opportunity to stay with the team through many changes in management and ownership, as the league grew and other teams and owners were brought in. The team later became known as the New York Red Bulls, and I became their head athletic trainer.

I used that position to educate more and more soccer enthusiasts about injuries and their prevention. Major League Soccer executives were so impressed with my knowledge and experience that they made me the league's medical coordinator in 2006. This position has afforded me the opportunity to work with not only our players but with soccer medicine colleagues from around the world. In any given week, I find myself consulting with professionals from soccer federations such as the English Premier League, Germany's Bundesliga, and Spain's La Liga. I regularly confer with U.S. players such as Tim Howard, Claudio Reyna, Tab Ramos, and Michael Bradley and have become a medical resource to the soccer community.

Along with my background and experience in the realm of professional soccer, I also own and operate JAG Physical Therapy, a private outpatient orthopedic sport physical therapy company with eight facilities in New Jersey and New York. At JAG Physical Therapy, I treat patients of all ages, shapes, and sizes, which allows me to utilize my expertise on not only the professional athlete, but on the youth athlete and weekend warrior as well. Whether you are playing your first game as a child, or are a businessman kicking the ball around with a few friends, injuries can occur. I work hard every day to get people back to 100% so they can continue doing what they love to do.

It is my hope that soccer enthusiasts will read this book and become much more versed in the soccer player's body and how it works during the game. Parents will understand how to seek treatment for the various injuries their children might suffer. Coaches will have a better understanding of how to prevent injuries during games and practices. Players will be better able to prevent nagging injuries and understand the rehabilitation process when it comes to more serious injuries, like chronic ankle instability or the very common anterior cruciate ligament tear. Readers will take away simple soccer conditioning, strengthening, flexibility, nutritional, and hydration techniques that will keep them playing the game instead of watching from the sidelines.

So let's move forward and learn. As my long-time friend and legendary American soccer coach Bob Bradley would say, "Let's get stuck in and compete."

# SOCCER INJURY PREVENTION AND TREATMENT

# CHAPTER ONE

# YOUTH INJURIES

As coaches and parents working with youth athletes, our primary concern should be their proper growth and development. No matter what stage of their career that athletes are in, growth and development is cyclical and there is always room for improvement. By varying training regimens and keeping them fun and interactive, we can be certain our children are learning what it takes to be successful not only on the field, but also in life.

Of course, we wouldn't have a topic for our book if it weren't for the injuries in soccer that are inevitable! Injuries specific to the youth athlete often arise from various growth patterns and disorders, combined with acute or chronic trauma. But even these youth-specific conditions can be easily managed with proper care and a logical treatment progression.

## SEVER'S DISEASE

Sever's disease, or calcaneal apophysitis, is a painful bone disorder resulting from inflammation in the calcaneal epiphyseal plate, or growth plate, in the heel. A growth plate is an area of growing tissue at the end of a developing bone. Over time, cartilage cells change into bone cells and the growth plates expand and join together, which is how bones grow.

The calcaneal epiphyseal plate is the growth center of the heel bone where the Achilles tendon attaches at the heel (see Figure 1.1). Sever's disease is a common cause of heel pain in growing kids, especially those who are very active. This condition typically arises during the growth spurts in the adolescent years—between the ages of 8 and 13 for girls, and 10 and 15 for boys. During these years, adolescents are experiencing rapid growth with immature bone transforming into fully matured bone. Sever's disease rarely occurs in older teenagers because the growth plate in the heel typically hardens by age 15.

**Mechanism of Injury**

During an adolescent growth spurt, the heel bone can grow faster than the leg muscles and tendons around it. This causes the muscles and tendons, especially the Achilles tendon or heel cord, to become very tight and to pull directly on the growth

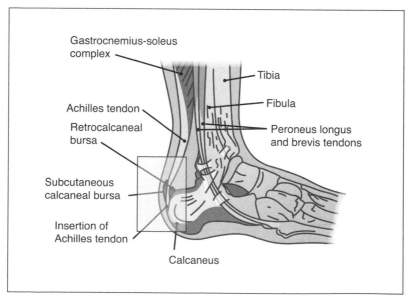

**Figure 1.1** Anatomy: Calcaneus with Achilles attachment.

plate in the calcaneus, or heel bone. This increase in stress and tension, which is exacerbated with activity, causes an irritation at the heel. Over time, repeated stress can damage the growth plate, causing the swelling, tenderness, and pain of Sever's disease.

Though Sever's disease can occur in any growing child, certain conditions, such as pronated feet that roll in at the ankle, flat or high arches, short leg syndrome (where one leg is shorter than the other), and childhood obesity may increase the chances of its development.

### Signs and Symptoms of Sever's Disease

The symptoms of Sever's disease are seen most often in the running athlete (which, of course, includes soccer). Complaints most often include heel pain, tightness, swelling, and sometimes bruising. The pain will increase with running and jumping activities, and may be exacerbated with a tight shoe or boot.

### Treatment of Sever's Disease

If Sever's disease is identified early on, treatment can be successful and will limit any long-term difficulties that might arise. Take note of when the athlete begins to complain of heel pain, so a doctor or physical therapist can assess how the symptoms are progressing.

The initial goal in the treatment of Sever's disease is pain relief through a decrease in inflammation. The best way to accomplish this is with the RICE protocol: Rest, Ice, Compression, and Elevation.

Icing at the heel is best done with an ice cup (see Figure 1.2), for approximately 15 minutes, four times per day. Once the initial inflammatory response has subsided, a flexibility program can be started for the Achilles tendon to limit the tension being placed on the growth plate. The goal is to increase the elasticity of the calf muscles and associated tendons that insert at the calcaneus (see Figure 1.3).

No treatment can change the course of a child's growth spurt, nor can we determine when growth spurts will begin and how long they will last. Should symptoms arise, they must simply be treated appropriately with rest and modified activity. Rest is

| RICE PROTOCOL | |
|---|---|
| Rest | Remove the stress. This means take a break from, change, or altogether stop any activity that increases pain or soreness. |
| Ice* | Three to four times per day, 15 min per session, remembering not to leave on too long to avoid potential damage to the skin. |
| Compression | Wrap the injured area with an elastic bandage to aide in limiting inflammation. |
| Elevation | Use pillows to elevate the injured area while sitting or lying down. Gravity will help to pull the inflammation back toward the core of the body. |

*A note about icing: With soft tissue tendon injuries, it is often more beneficial to administer an ice massage rather than to simply lay a bag of ice or frozen peas over the injured area. Freeze water in a Dixie cup, peel away the excess paper and use the cup to massage the area. The massaging action will decrease the inflammation and pain in the area at a more efficient rate.

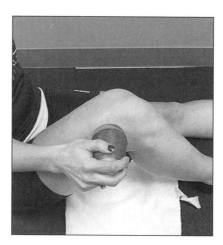

**Figure 1.2** Ice cup massage: A good way to target a superficial tissue with cryotherapy. Simply freeze a half-filled wax paper cup with water, peel back the excess and apply the ice directly to the skin in a gentle circular pattern for 10 minutes, or until the skin is sufficiently numb.

important to the resolution of Sever's disease, so pressure on the heel bone can be relieved. Athletes will often have to sit out for a period of time to allow the pain and swelling to subside. In severe

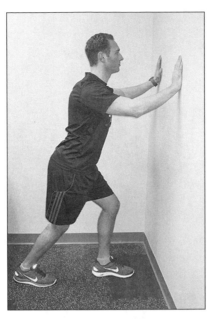

**Figure 1.3** Calf stretch: Keeping your heel firmly planted on the floor, step forward with your opposite foot and apply a gentle stretch to your calf.

cases, doctors may even choose to immobilize the foot in a cast or boot to allow for healing (see Figure 1.4). After the athlete can walk without pain, a good protocol to improve the strength and flexibility of the foot and heel cord are important for successful outcomes.

After enough time has passed to restore strength and flexibility, we can begin functional and sport-specific activity to physically prepare the athlete for a partial return to sport. In the beginning, the athlete can participate at a 50% to 75% level in order to keep them involved while limiting the trauma to the heel. For this athlete, low-impact soccer drills and skills are better than more stressful long runs.

Remember, do not neglect the foot! Elasticity within the plantar fascia can also be helpful in curbing the symptoms of Sever's disease by dispersing the ground reaction forces experienced at the heel and above. Simple stretching is beneficial, deep-tissue massage is even better and can be done by rolling the foot on a firm ball to break up any adhesions (see Figure 1.5). This same method can and should be done at the calf muscle belly.

The soccer player, based on the type and fit of the soccer boot, may also want to protect the area with an arch support or heel lift to decrease direct trauma to an already sensitive area.

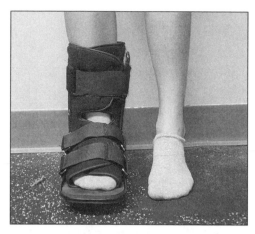

**Figure 1.4** A CAM (controlled ankle movement) boot immobilizes the foot and controls ankle motion to allow for healing while at the same time allowing the athlete to bear weight and be ambulatory.

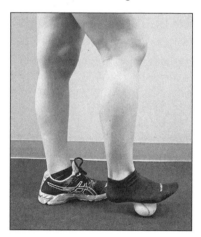

**Figure 1.5** Myofascial tissue release: A deep tissue massage for the plantar fascia using a tennis or golf ball. Place tolerable pressure through the bottom of your foot onto the ball, and gently roll forward and backwards on the ball.

## OSGOOD–SCHLATTER'S DISEASE

Osgood–Schlatter's disease is similar to Sever's disease, but occurs at the knee joint rather than at the heel. Specifically, pain and inflammation occurs at the proximal tibia where the quadriceps tendon inserts into the bone, at the bony protuberance below the knee cap (see Figure 1.6). This protuberance is more prominent in some individuals, and is often the result of the same type of force reaction that defines Sever's disease. In general, a tight quadriceps tendon pulls on the growth plate during running and jumping activities. When combined with rapid growth spurts in adolescent athletes, Osgood–Schlatter's disease can result. Most often, it only affects one knee, and is more prevalent in boys than in girls. It is relatively common, occurring in about one of every five youth athletes.

### Signs and Symptoms of Osgood–Schlatter's Disease

Swelling and inflammation exists directly at the site of trauma, often with point tenderness. A visible, painful bump may develop just below the knee joint at the proximal tibia. The muscles surrounding the knee, including the hamstring and quadriceps, may be tight. Adults who experienced Osgood–Schlatter as adolescents may still have a visibly enlarged bone protuberance. This symptom can remain, and must be managed throughout an athlete's career.

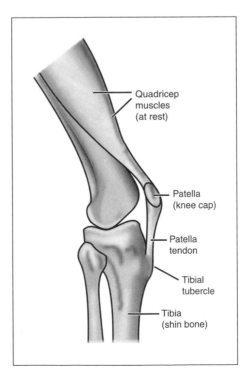

Quadricep
muscles
(at rest)

Patella
(knee cap)

Patella
tendon

Tibial
tubercle

Tibia
(shin bone)

**Figure 1.6** Anatomy: Tibia tubercule with quad attachment.

## Treatment of Osgood–Schlatter's Disease

Symptoms of Osgood–Schlatter's disease can be acutely exacerbated with activity, so there needs to be a period of RICE to reduce pain and swelling at the knee. After inflammation is controlled, a program can begin to increase elasticity in the surrounding musculature (see Figure 1.7). A good quadriceps-strengthening protocol should be included, beginning with muscle-setting exercises done on a table, such as quad sets, and advancing to include closed kinetic chain exercises (in which the limb is in contact with either the ground or another stable surface, such as squats or lunges). Avoiding open kinetic chain activities (when the limb is not in contact with the ground or any other stable surface and is free to move, such as a leg extension) will also help with this injury, since these exercises often increase the symptoms. Anti-inflammatory drugs, or nonsteroidal anti-inflammatory drugs (NSAIDs), may be warranted, depending on the severity of pain and level of dysfunction.

As the athlete's pain decreases and elasticity increases, he or she can gradually be returned back to play. Once again, while we cannot change the growth pattern of the child, we can limit

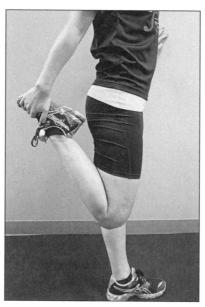

**Figure 1.7** Standing quad stretch: Standing with support, bend the knee, grab the foot and pull upward, keeping the hips open and extended. Try not to bend at the hip.

symptoms of Osgood–Schlatter's disease by removing activities that irritate the area. If the athlete feels good enough for passing and dribbling drills and strengthening exercises, but running uphill sprints exacerbates the pain, coaches need to work with the athlete to make accommodations within the training protocol. The goal is to keep the athlete on the field, not sitting on the sideline because of a need to run sprints after practice. It is important for parents, athletes, and coaches to work together for proper management of the signs and symptoms of Osgood–Schlatter's disease, and to keep the athlete under the care of a physical therapist or athletic trainer.

## PATELLOFEMORAL SYNDROME

Patellofemoral syndrome is an overuse injury seen in youth athletes, caused by friction on the cartilage under the patella, or kneecap. This causes a softening, roughening, or general degeneration of the cartilage under the kneecap, known as chondromalacia.

### Mechanism of Injury

Typically, the patella tracks in a straight line in the trochlear groove at the center of the thigh bone, and pressure is spread over the widest possible area. If the patella is tilted or slides outside of this groove, pressure is uneven and can irritate the cartilage under the patella. Improper tracking of the kneecap can be caused by a variety of pre-existing conditions, including flat feet, knock-knees, or weakness of the hip and thigh muscles. This disorder often affects females more than males, due to the widening of the pelvis during the adolescent years. The quadriceps tendon will pull more laterally on the patella, which causes the female adolescent athlete to be predisposed for patellar subluxation, which can cause biological changes at the knee. One such change is chronic weakness of the vastus medialis obliquus (VMO) muscle, which is the quadriceps muscle on the inside of the thigh. This muscle provides stability to the knee, and when weakened can contribute to incorrect tracking of the patella.

Repeated subluxation of the patella, or trauma to the posterior side of the patella (the side that articulates with the trochlear groove of the femur), also causes a rubbing or grinding of the cartilage behind the knee cap, which has degenerative effects over time.

## Signs and Symptoms of Patellofemoral Syndrome

The biomechanical deviation of the kneecap in patellofemoral syndrome causes an inflammatory response, resulting in pain and swelling behind the kneecap. It can also cause compensatory changes in the gait pattern. Pain may be aggravated by activity, and also by long periods of sitting with the knees in a moderately bent position; this is known as the "theater" or "movie-goers" sign of patellofemoral syndrome. The athlete may also complain of tightness or a feeling of fullness at the front of the knee. Patellofemoral syndrome does not always cause crippling pain, but it can lead to debilitating degenerative changes over time.

## Treatment of Patellofemoral Syndrome

Patellofemoral syndrome is something most players can deal with and will attempt to play through, if their pain is mostly tolerable. However, if not properly managed, patellofemoral syndrome can progress into a more severe injury that may require surgical intervention, such as a fissuring or fracturing of the patella.

Initially, a RICE protocol is essential to limit the inflammation caused by patellofemoral syndrome. A physician may elect to prescribe anti-inflammatory drugs, or NSAIDs. Beyond immediate treatment to manage pain and inflammation, it is essential to change the biomechanics of the knee in order to correct the cause of this syndrome.

It's important to get the VMO to fire in the proper sequence, and to make it strong enough so it pulls the kneecap in the proper direction (see Figure 1.8). The simplest way to do this is through isolation, through muscle-setting exercises such as quad sets, straight leg raises, adductor leg raises, and standing terminal knee extensions (see Figure 1.9). Strengthening the abductor and

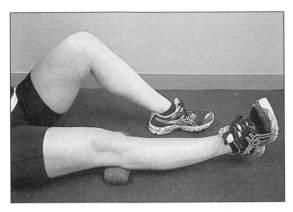

**Figure 1.8** Quad set: Muscle-setting exercise to strengthen the quad and regain neuromuscular control. Place a bolster behind the knee and firmly contract the quadriceps, elevating the heel off the floor or table.

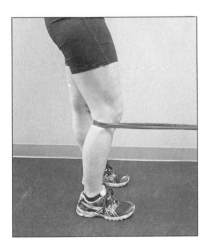

**Figure 1.9** TKE (terminal knee extension): This closed kinetic chain, quadriceps-strengthening exercise works on the final 30 degrees of range of motion with band resistance. Slightly bend your knee, tracking your toes, and extend to just before a full lock-out position.

hip extensor muscles helps to decrease the incidence of patellofemoral syndrome.

If not treated appropriately, patellofemoral syndrome can result in more serious issues that require surgical intervention.

# CHAPTER TWO

# OVERUSE INJURIES

In this chapter we will be discussing overuse injuries in soccer, but before we continue, it is important to understand the difference between an acute injury and an overuse injury.

Acute injuries are typically the result of a single, traumatic event, such as a collision or fall, and include fractures, sprains, and dislocations. If you "hear a pop" or "feel a snap," you have likely suffered an acute injury. Overuse injuries are much more subtle and their cause often cannot be traced to a specific moment. They happen over time, and are the result of repetitive micro-trauma to the bones, tendons, and joints.

When we exercise, bones, muscles, tendons, and ligaments get stronger as they are broken down during activity and then built back up during recovery. But if the rebuilding of the tissue cannot keep up with the breaking down of the tissue, injury occurs.

As we all know, soccer is an action sport that includes a lot of repetitive movements, such as running, cutting, and kicking. The specific forces placed on a soccer athlete often lead to chronic overuse injuries, primarily of the lower extremities—the feet, knees, and hips. The following is a discussion of some of these commonly seen injuries.

## ACHILLES TENDINITIS

The single structure known as the Achilles tendon takes the two calf muscles—the gastrocnemius and soleus—and combines them into the tendon, connecting at the back of the heel, or calcaneus (see Figure 2.1).

When we're talking about tendinitis, we're discussing a tendon that is swollen or undergoing an inflammatory response. During this process, damaged tissue cells release chemicals that cause blood vessels to leak fluid into the tissue, causing swelling.

In normal, healthy tissue, the tendon and the sheath slide and glide naturally with each other. Due to repetitive actions, or even a change in intensity, the fluid released by the inflammatory response essentially takes up space within the tendon sheath, which increases the amount of friction between the tendon and the sheath. Typically, an athlete will feel some pain or discomfort when this occurs, and if the athlete continues to stress the area by attempting to play through it, the inflammation will increase, leading to less and less space within the tendon sheath.

It is important to note the potential progression with continued use. The building effect of degenerative inflammation will damage the tissue, and lead to worsening degrees of tendinitis. All types of tendinitis can vary in severity from Stage I to Stage IV.

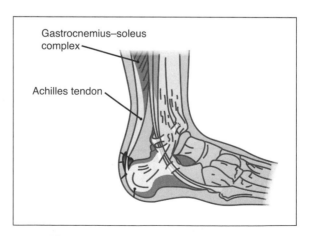

Gastrocnemius–soleus complex

Achilles tendon

**Figure 2.1** Anatomy: Achilles tendon.

### Stages of Tendinitis

**Stage I.** Pain after activity. Normal function. No gait changes; normal walking and running.

**Stage II.** Pain during and after activity. Soccer athlete can still participate, because warming up increases circulation and masks pain. The athlete may feel good for a short period, but there is no tendon healing.

**Stage III.** Prolonged pain during and after activity. Antalgic, or shortened, gait. The athlete cannot perform any activity at a satisfactory level.

**Stage IV.** Actual tearing of tendon, with the possibility of having a surgical intervention.

### Signs and Symptoms of Achilles Tendinitis

Usually, the soccer player will complain about tightness or pain in the Achilles area, mostly in the mornings when first getting out of bed and putting a foot to the floor. Walking loosens this up, but stationary periods lead to tightness and pain.

The soccer player will also, as he or she continues to play, start to feel a severe pain along the Achilles tendon, which, if not treated appropriately, can lead to a tear. A tear of the Achilles tendon is a very serious injury that requires surgery and up to a year of rehabilitation. Simple tendinitis is much easier to fix, so it is important to tend to it as quickly as possible.

The area around the Achilles tendon may also be visibly swollen, with swelling increasing throughout the day or during activity.

### Prevention of Achilles Tendinitis

There are simple ways to prevent the onset of Achilles tendinitis, as long as the soccer player understands a true progression of training. Simply speaking, you cannot do too much, too quickly. A gradual progression from low to high intensity and frequency as certain plateaus are achieved will allow for proper physiological adaptations to occur at a more natural rate.

The human body is amazing and can adapt to almost any environment imaginable. Through soccer training, we are essentially molding our bodies into the perfect tool to succeed at our sport.

Close your eyes and picture Olympic weightlifters. Now, imagine all of the strength training and hours spent perfecting their technique to mold their bodies into the ultimate lifting machine. Through their specific training regimen, their bodies have adapted to the external stimuli of moving heavy weight.

Of course, none of this happens overnight. Regardless of what sport we play, we must put in the training and practice hours necessary to improve our acumen for that given skill set. By gradually increasing our loads and intensity, we allow for our body to recover and adapt at a more natural rate. We can now move on to more physically demanding activities as we build upon our foundation, striving to be the ultimate soccer player.

Other preventive measures would be ensuring that shoes fit properly, warming up properly before activity, and maintaining flexibility through various stretching techniques and deep-tissue massage (see Figure 2.2).

Also, a soccer athlete should try not to change surfaces continuously throughout their training regimen, meaning they should not switch often between playing on concrete and playing on turf or grass.

### Treatment of Achilles Tendinitis

Achilles tendinitis is very treatable. Central to proper treatment of tendinitis is identifying the cause of the problem. Some examples might include:

- Change of intensity
- A muscle not properly warmed up or stretched prior to activity
- Training surface changes (hard and soft)
- Running too hard or too much
- Continual, repetitive jumping and cutting
- Changing shoes, ill-fitting shoes, or shoes that are not supportive

By limiting or removing the cause, we can slow down or reverse the inflammatory response and cure the tendinitis.

Before treating a soccer athlete, it is important to recognize the way the athlete is walking. Is there a noticeable limp? Does the

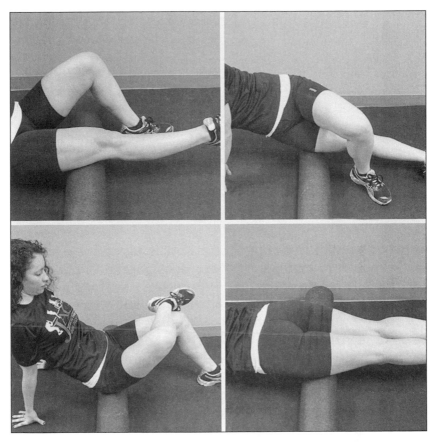

**Figure 2.2** Foam roller: The foam roller allows you to utilize your own body weight to apply pressure to different tissues of the body by rolling across the length of the muscle and providing a deep tissue massage. Usually done for one to two minutes per muscle group.

athlete favor one side over the other? Is the athlete having difficulty decelerating or accelerating, or jumping or planting?

If the answer to any of those questions is "yes," then the tendon likely has some level of inflammation. At this point the player should RICE it! (see chart on page 4).

If pain is severe, it is advisable at this point to see a doctor for an evaluation and assessment for the direction of care. While Achilles tendinitis does not usually require surgical intervention, it can sometimes benefit from immobilization in a boot or cast to limit motion of the foot and ankle. But if proper attention is paid to the injury in its early stages, it can be handled before it progresses to an aggressive stage.

If the Achilles tendinitis is only causing soreness and pain, and is not affecting the athlete's gait or performance, I recommend:

- Heel lifts bilaterally (in both shoes), to raise the heel and alleviate tension in the Achilles and calf
- A good warm-up and stretching routine
- Practice modification

As the inflammation surrounding the tendon decreases, the pain will go away. As the player starts to feel less pain and tightness in the area, based on the increased flexibility and the treatment suggested, there should be a modified progression for a return to play.

With Achilles tendinitis, athletes often have a lot of success if they return to training at 50% of their normal level of activity. This means simply cutting the athlete's workload in half; if the team is doing 10 sprints, the athlete would do 5. If they're practicing for an hour, the injured athlete would practice for 30 minutes. If successful, the workload builds gradually up to 75%, 80%, and eventually 100%. If the tendinitis becomes more exaggerated, the athlete should seek appropriate medical care in the form of a good physical therapist or athletic trainer.

In the clinic, we will be able to use different types of modalities and devices to increase circulation to the tendon, which will assist in decreasing the swelling and inflammation.

The sports medicine professional will then progress with different massage and stretching techniques. When adequate time has been allowed for healing of the area, a progression of therapeutic exercises will assist in safely returning the athlete's strength and coordination.

Once a solid foundation is laid, the athlete will be able to progress to functional, sport-specific exercises, including running, jumping, backpedaling, and side-shuffling. As the foundation increases, more general soccer skills can be introduced. Eventually, the athlete can return to on-field activities and progress to a full return to practice.

Too many times in my career, I have seen athletes with Achilles tendinitis return to play too quickly. While an adequate course of treatment could effectively eliminate the injury, the athlete is instead plagued by the injury throughout the season, and often throughout a career. I've also seen athletes hurt themselves worse by tearing their Achilles, which puts them on the sidelines for an entire season, simply because they didn't take the time to properly treat their initial injury.

As we all know, in order to continue playing the game we love, we must take the necessary steps at staying healthy and in the game.

## PATELLAR TENDINITIS

As we move up the soccer player's leg, we come to the almighty knee. Soccer inherently has a high rate of injury to the lower extremities, and the knee specifically accounts for a large portion of those injuries.

A common chronic injury of the knee is patellar tendinitis, which develops over time from repeated flexion and extension of the knee. Inflammation builds up just below the kneecap, directly over the patellar tendon. This tendon is responsible for controlling the action of the four large quadriceps muscles, and attaches to the lower leg bone, or tibia, at the tibial tubercle, which is the prominent bony aspect at the top of the shin, about two inches below the knee cap.

The repetitive actions of running, jumping, and kicking in soccer cause friction within the patellar tendon and tendon sheath. This friction inevitably causes an inflammatory process that results in swelling directly over the patellar tendon. This makes the knee feel very tight and swollen. The athlete will have difficulty going up and down stairs, getting in and out of cars, running for long periods of time (especially uphill and downhill), jumping repetitively, and of course, kicking the ball!

Patellar tendinitis is often referred to as *jumper's knee*. As with all types of tendinitis, classifications range in severity from Stage I to Stage IV (see page 15 for the stages of tendinitis).

### Prevention of Patellar Tendinitis

There are some easy ways to prevent and treat patellar tendinitis. For starters, wear appropriate footwear for the soccer surface: turf shoes for turf, cleats for grass, and flats for indoor.

**Flexibility:** Maintaining the flexibility of the patellar tendon prevents the onset of patellar tendinitis. In Figures 1.6 and 5.3, we show two simple quadriceps stretches, to be completed in 15-second intervals for three sets, before and after both training and games. Along with this static stretching, athletes should perform a dynamic warm-up to increase blood flow to the area. As a general rule, athletes are properly warmed up once they break a sweat, and should be sweating prior to beginning any soccer-related training activity.

**Weakness:** Despite an athlete's ability to perform on the training field, the quadriceps muscles can be too weak for soccer actions. This is especially prevalent in the adolescent female, and it is important for soccer athletes to strengthen the surrounding musculature of the ankle, knee, and hip joints. Most patellar tendinitis injuries can be limited with a good quad-strengthening routine that includes plyometrics, functional training, and a flexibility component. Each of these modalities should be introduced in a progression throughout the season.

### Treatment of Patellar Tendinitis

Of course, early intervention is the best treatment available (outside of prevention). Athletes must seek the help of a sports medicine professional immediately after they begin to feel discomfort, especially if their gait pattern has changed. The sports medicine professional will be able to identify and limit the cause of the discomfort and alleviate symptoms. Such factors as intensity of training and the amount of repetitive actions such as running, jumping, and kicking will be taken into consideration. It is likely that a modification of practice and game schedules will be necessary. When caught early, patellar tendinitis is easily treated, but again, it can plague the athlete for a long period of time if not taken care of appropriately and in a timely manner.

If pain and swelling have just begun, they can be easily treated with the RICE protocol (see chart on page 4) and the stretching exercises shown in this chapter.

If the patellar tendinitis is more aggressive and has changed the gait pattern, a normal treatment protocol will include modification of practice, modification of games, utilization of physical therapy modalities, hands-on massage, icing, strengthening, flexibility, progression of functional strengthening (see Figure 2.3), progression of

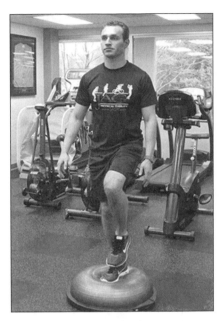

**Figure 2.3** Bosu balance exercise: While maintaining a stable ankle, knee and hip, balance on one leg for 30 seconds. Repeat three times. Variation. Include a ball toss to further improve balance.

sport-specific return-to-play exercises, and ultimately, a returning to the field of play.

As suggested many times before, you cannot jump from the treatment table directly to the field. There should be a good opportunity to train for at least a full week before returning back to any game.

Many people wait too long to treat their patellar tendinitis, or ignore it altogether, and it causes a degeneration of the tendon. Sometimes, the tendon can be so badly damaged that a surgeon must intervene, using steroid or platelet-rich plasma injections or scrapings to repair or remove the degenerative tendon, all with various success rates. The goal of any soccer player with patellar tendinitis should be to treat it early and stay on the field.

## IT BAND SYNDROME

Continuing up the soccer athlete's leg, we come to the ilio-tibial (IT) band. Most people that have pain consistent with an IT band dysfunction usually complain of lateral (outside) knee pain. But most people don't realize that the IT band originates as the tensor fascia lata (TFL) muscle (not to be confused with your favorite Starbucks beverage!) at the outside of the hip (ilium), runs along the lateral quadriceps muscle (vastus lateralis), and inserts just below the knee joint line on the tibia.

IT band syndrome (ITBS) is most commonly caused by friction between the distal IT band and the lateral femoral epicondyle, which is the bump on the outside of the knee. It is a very common injury associated with running athletes, such as the soccer player, and is one of the leading causes of lateral knee pain. The tightness distending from the lateral quadricep muscle, the vastus lateralis, closes the available space between the bone and tendon, leading to increased friction while flexing and extending the knee.

Since this tendon crosses two joints, the level of debilitation can cause changes in the function of both the hip and knee when walking or running. Deviations from the normal gait pattern can lead to compensatory pain in other joints above or below the affected area.

From a mechanical perspective, this musculotendinous complex is crucial to the stabilization of the knee during running. With the knee in a flexed position, the IT band sits behind the femur (the large upper leg bone) and passes to the front of the femur during knee extension; that is, the IT band moves with each stride, and the friction leads to the body's inflammatory response.

ITBS symptoms can range from a stiff joint to swelling or thickening along the entire IT band (not just around the knee). Some people describe the sensation as a stinging, burning, or numbness around the knee joint, most often on the lateral side. Depending on the severity of dysfunction, this sensation can extend from the knee all the way up to the hip.

As with any inflammatory process, pain usually begins as mild discomfort after activity and becomes more intense over time. The pain is usually felt when the foot hits the ground, and will persist in aggravation after activity. The progression of pain is typically noticed before or after activity, when moving from sitting to standing or walking up and down stairs. When pain is present during normal daily activities, it is time to begin treatment to alleviate symptoms.

### Prevention of IT Band Syndrome

IT band syndrome is an overuse injury, but there are some factors that can contribute to its acceleration. If an athlete trains on different levels of surface, be it downhill, uphill, or on an embankment, the body must adjust. Take a look at your street. Does it slope uphill or downhill? Or is the center of the road higher than the shoulder of the road? Consistently running the same trail or pattern will likely lead to imbalances from compensatory movements.

Muscular imbalances could be another cause of ITBS. Analysis of the lateral versus medial quadriceps muscles will likely point to an overactive lateralis, causing tightness around the IT band. Weak hip adductors can also contribute to IT band pain. A physical therapist can teach the patient how to strengthen the entire quad grouping and help the muscles to fire at a more optimal rate.

Poor training habits can also contribute to the injury. Athlete's need to warm up and cool down properly, and should not do too much, too fast, too soon.

Maintaining the flexibility of the IT band with stretching (see Figure 2.4) and the aid of a foam roller can help to prevent the onset of IT band syndrome.

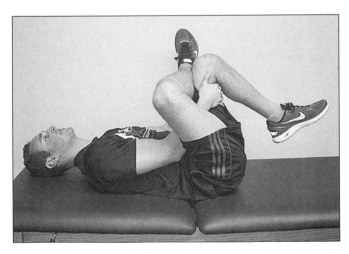

**Figure 2.4** Piriformis stretch: While in a seated position, place the right foot over the left knee, making a figure 4. Lie back and flex the left hip up toward your chest, grabbing the left thigh for support. The stretch should be felt in the right buttocks. Repeat on the opposite side.

**Treatment of IT Band Syndrome**

It is important to remember that IT band syndrome isn't just an overuse knee injury, due to its origin at the hip. Treatment should target the joints both above and below the TFL, that is, the knee and hip, and should also address the vastus lateralis muscle.

Since the primary mechanism leading to ITBS is continual flexing and extending of the knee, it is important to limit or remove completely this causal factor. Simply, take a few days off!

As with almost any injury, the first step in treating ITBS is to RICE to reduce pain and inflammation (see chart on page 4). In addition, any tight tendon should be put through a daily stretching routine to increase its internal flexibility. If proper attention is paid to ITBS at its onset, it can be managed easily. But again, if the injury has progressed to the point where the athlete is experiencing pain with each step, along with gait changes, it is advisable to seek the attention of a medical professional.

An accomplished practitioner will utilize appropriate therapeutic modalities to increase circulation and decrease the inflammatory process of the fascial tissue of the tendon. As pliability of the tissue is restored, flexibility will increase and the downward pressure of the tendon on the knee will dissipate.

As the soccer player's symptoms begin to decrease, it is now appropriate for the physical therapist or athletic trainer to use massage, increase strengthening techniques, and ultimately start to progress the athlete to more functional, sport-specific exercises. As long as the soccer player is responding well to therapy, he or she can start to do some light playing, so long as he or she follows a good progression to return to play.

## TIBIAL STRESS REACTIONS (STRESS FRACTURES AND SHIN SPLINTS)

Another common overuse injury for running athletes is the stress fracture, which is a hairline crack in the bone caused by the repetitive application of force. In the 19th century, stress fractures were known as "military" or "march" fractures, diagnosed in Prussian soldiers after repetitive marching. Soccer players may not be soldiers or marathoners, but they do cover up to six miles in a typical match. In soccer athletes, stress fractures most often occur in the shin bone or tibia (see Figure 2.5), which, despite being a relatively small bone, carries 90% of the body's weight.

While most stress fractures occur when fatigued muscles can't absorb the shock of repeated impact and subsequently transfer the stress of the load to the bone, some can also arise through an innate weakness in the bone, often due to conditions such as osteoporosis.

Our bones are made up of living, breathing tissue, and are not a stale or stagnant part of our bodies. With repetitive trauma, we are constantly breaking down our bone cells. When we rest, we give our bodies a chance to rebuild the damaged tissue so it does not break down completely.

Stress fractures typically result as a progression of medial tibial stress syndrome, or shin splints. Shin splints occur when the muscle pulls away from its attachment to the tibia. When the

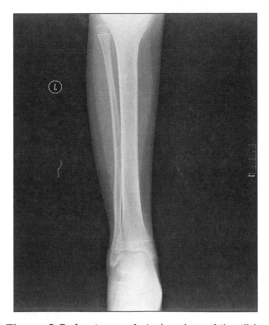

**Figure 2.5** Anatomy: Anterior view of the tibia.

muscle is not there as an absorption tool, the bone becomes the primary absorber of force.

Stress fractures in the bone occur when there is an imbalance between how much we are breaking down and how much we are rebuilding on a daily basis. If we break down more than we rebuild, the structure will ultimately fail.

### Signs and Symptoms of Tibial Stress Reactions

A tibial stress reaction is felt in the lower part of the shin, primarily on the medial (inner) side. Early onset pain is generally noticed during activity, and progresses to bouts of pain after activity. Often, a hot spot or tender spot will develop along the shin, and will be felt by the athlete when palpating along the length of the bone.

The only true way for a medical professional to diagnose shin splints or a stress fracture is with either an x-ray, bone scan, or MRI. If the fracture is large enough to be seen on an x-ray, the athlete will have been in considerable pain for a long time. Often, x-rays can identify evidence of bone healing, indicative of a stress reaction.

### Causes of Tibial Stress Reactions

Some of the causes of a stress fracture can be poor biomechanics, flat feet or fallen arches, inflexible or weak muscles (as I keep saying, too much too soon!), improper shoes, or training and playing excessively on hard surfaces.

Stress fractures are more often seen in female athletes, when an intensive training program is combined with a poor diet and naturally lower calcium levels. This is known as the female athlete triad. Contributing factors may be an eating disorder, osteoporosis, or dysmenorrhea (pain during menstruation) or amenorrhea (absence of a menstrual period in a woman of reproductive age).

Preventing stress fractures, then, also relies on the importance of a well-balanced diet, with the inclusion of vitamin D, and making sure the athletes train with the appropriate equipment.

## Treatment of Tibial Stress Reactions

There are many different schools of thought about treating stress fractures in the sports medicine world. I believe if you continue to run on a small fracture, it will eventually develop into a full fracture, which will effectively put you on the sideline for 8 to 10 weeks.

Again, we go back to early recognition. It is important to identifying a possible stress reaction as soon as possible, and realize that everybody recovers differently. Because of the difficulty in differentiating between a stress fracture and a shin splint, it is a good idea to stop activity and see a health care professional as soon as shin pain is felt.

With shin splints and stress fractures in the lower leg, it is also important to remember that rest may not only mean taking a break from running and playing soccer. The standing and walking we do to complete normal, daily activities can also often be too much for a bone that has been stressed.

It may be necessary to put the athlete in a walking boot, air cast, or full lower leg air cast for 4 to 8 weeks, and up to 16 to 20 weeks if the injury progresses to a full fracture.

Whether the injury requires immobilization or not, it is important that the athlete be pain-free prior to beginning any type of strengthening or aerobic activity.

Once pain-free, phase one of recovery is to restore range of motion (see Figure 2.6). The ankle joint must have a full range of motion before functional training can begin. In addition, good flexibility of the lower leg muscles will help long term by allowing for more shock absorption in the lower extremity during running and training (see Figure 2.7).

Phase two, which can coincide with phase one, is to begin low-level, low-impact strengthening. This may include four-way ankle exercises for the shin, ankle, and foot muscles, including the gastrocnemius–soleus complex and anterior tibialis (see Figure 2.8).

Finally, phase three of rehab will progress the athlete into functional and full weight-bearing activities (see Figure 2.9). As with any injury, there is no direct route from the training table back to the field. Athletes must recover their general fitness, then gradually progress to a full return to play.

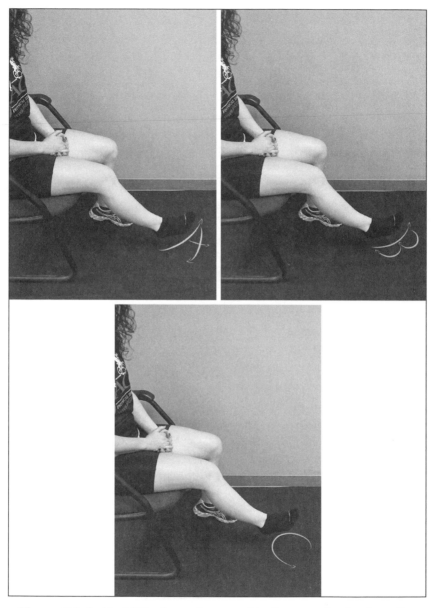

**Figure 2.6** Ankle ABCs: A good range of motion exercise to stress the multiplanar motion of the foot and ankle. Simply write the ABCs in the air with the big toe.

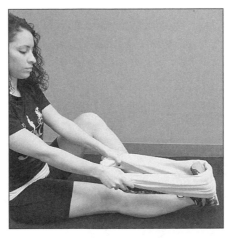

**Figure 2.7** Towel stretch: While sitting upright, place a towel around the toes and pull them up toward the shin. Hold for 30 seconds and repeat three times. This is a good athlete-controlled Achilles stretch to use after an acute injury.

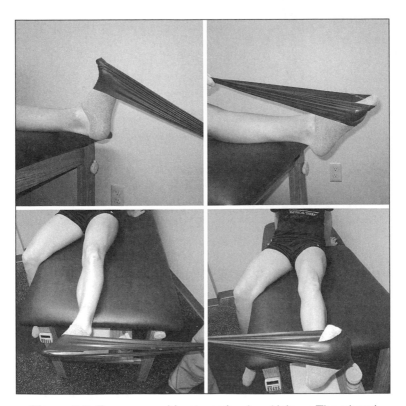

**Figure 2.8** Four-way ankle strengthening: Using a Theraband as resistance, complete the following four motions (dorsiflexion, plantarflexion, inversion, and eversion) for three sets of ten reps each.

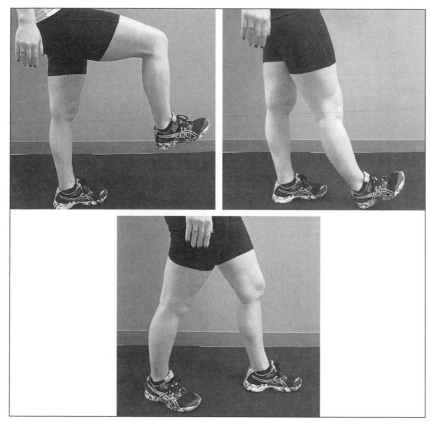

**Figure 2.9** Functional walks: Make sure you have a stable base of support. Elevate the knee, flexing at the hip. Step down, placing the heel on the ground first. Step through and repeat on the opposite side. Over-exaggerate the motion for maximum benefit.

## BURSITIS

The last of the overuse injuries we will discuss is bursitis. Between our muscles, tendons, and bones are small bursal sacs of synovial fluid, which is the body's lubricant. These sacs act as cushions and help joints move more fluidly by reducing friction between tendons and bones (see Figure 2.10).

Bursa sacs in any joint can become inflamed, but inflammation will generally occur in response to specific motions that are repeated over time. A simple way to imagine this is to picture stretching a rubber band and rubbing it against the side of a desk. The rubber band will eventually tear from the friction that

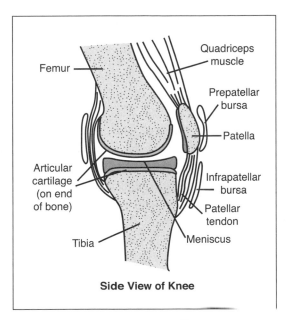

**Figure 2.10** Anatomy: Bursa sac.

is generated. Now imagine placing a small bladder of liquid in between the rubber band and the desk. This would decrease the amount of friction generated between the desk and the band (or bone and tendon) by acting as a buffer between the two surfaces. But with repeated trauma, even the bursa sac can become inflamed.

Another factor to take into account is the internal extensibility, or flexibility, of the tendon, or the tendon's ability to be stretched. As we continue with our rubber band example, think about the different types of bands. Some are short and thick and have little extensibility, while others are long and thin and have greater extensibility.

When these bursa sacs become inflamed, it causes pain and stiffness with simple flexion and extension. Depending on the severity, there may be a huge amount of inflammation around the joint. As you can imagine, as running athletes, soccer players usually get bursitis in their legs! The most common types of bursitis in soccer players are:

- Prepatellar, at the front of the knee
- Infrapatellar, below your kneecap
- Trochanteric, at the hip bone

- Achilles, at the calf tendon
- Iliopsoas, at the front of the hip
- Ischial, at the buttocks (those two bones you sit on all day long)

Underlying factors such as rheumatoid arthritis can contribute to bursitis, but it is most commonly a result of overuse. It can also result from trauma from a fall, most commonly in the buttocks, hip, or knee. As with any fluid-filled sac, a direct blow to the bursa has the ability to rupture the bursa. When this happens, there is generally a large amount of extra-articular swelling, or swelling outside the joint. Often, the joint itself is not maximally inhibited, and much of the joint's function remains intact.

If an infection is suspected, the athlete must be examined by a physician immediately for an appropriate diagnosis. Some common signs and symptoms of an infected bursa sac include:

- Erythema (redness)
- Swelling
- Giving off heat, or warm to the touch
- Increased pain and tenderness

Advanced bursitis results in a very red, swollen, stiff, painful joint. Some patients have even described it as "a big ball of redness."

**Prevention of Bursitis**

By looking at the way the forces are distributed across the tendon, bursa, and bone, we can define ways to limit the amount of force and friction generated among these tissues. By increasing the flexibility of the surrounding musculature, we can decrease the amount of pressure generated over time with repetitive actions.

**Treatment of Bursitis**

Throughout the therapeutic process, the goal is to decrease the inflammation of the bursa, while increasing the flexibility of the tendon. As the inflammation of the bursa decreases, the stiffness in the joint will also decrease.

Bursitis will usually resolve in 7 to 10 days with good therapeutic management, and the athlete can return to sport quite rapidly as long as swelling around the joint has been eliminated.

If a physician suspects a potential infection, he or she may prescribe an antibiotic. If the bursitis becomes a chronic issue, the physician may perform an aspiration, which is the physical removal of the fluid with a syringe. In severe cases, the inflamed or infected bursa may also be removed surgically. If this course of action is needed, it will likely lead to more problems down the road, especially for the running athlete, possibly involving a surgical tendon repair.

Once again, a minor problem of inflexibility can develop into a deeper issue involving multiple tissues if left untreated. In order to achieve every soccer player's goal of staying on the field, early intervention is key!

# CHAPTER THREE

# FOOT AND ANKLE INJURIES

As most soccer players understand from personal experience, the area of the body with the highest incidence of injury is the foot and ankle. These are the soccer player's refined tools, and they require much maintenance over the career span of any athlete. In this chapter, we will discuss some of the most commonly suffered foot and ankle injuries, which regularly sideline soccer players across the world.

## ANATOMICAL MAKEUP OF THE ANKLE JOINT

Looking at the anatomical makeup of the ankle joint, it is essential to define the bony structures first, so we can define the position of instability. The ankle mortise is the joint made up of the distal tibia, fibula, and talus bones. Structurally, the tibia is our primary weight-bearing bone, through which ground forces are transmitted with each step. The fibula is a source of attachment for multiple ligaments, muscles, and tendons to extend off of and create action at the foot and ankle. Seated within these two structures (see Figure 3.1) is the talus. The talus is a saddle-shaped bone with the primary functions of dorsi- and plantar-flexion, or the pointing and flexing of the foot.

Lateral ankle sprains, when the foot rolls inward, are more common than medial ankle sprains, when the foot rolls outward. The fibula, the bone on the outside of the ankle, is longer than the tibia, the bone on the inside of the ankle, and the foot is subsequently more inclined to turn inward than outward. When the foot is pointed, the shape of the talus bone also creates an instability in which the foot is more likely to roll inward than outward. Conversely, when the ankle is flexed, it is in its most stable position. Athletic trainers will tape and brace ankles in a flexed position in an attempt at maintaining as much stability as possible.

When foot and ankle injuries occur on the soccer field, the foot and ankle will roll, or invert, toward the midline of the body. The tendons and ligaments that maintain stability on the outside, or lateral aspect, of the foot and ankle will overstretch, sometimes past the breaking point of their internal tensile strength.

The most commonly injured lateral ligaments are the anterior talofibular ligament (ATFL), the posterior talofibular ligament (PTFL), and the calcaneofibular ligament (CFL). All three originate from the most distal portion of the fibula, but insert at different places: the ATFL connects to the front of the talus bone at the top

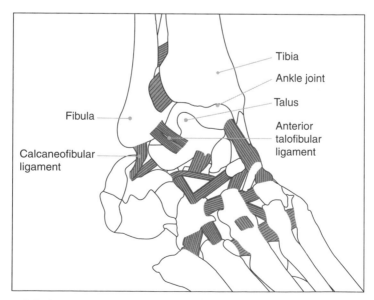

**Figure 3.1** Anatomy: Anterior view of ankle bones (tibia, fibula, and talus), and ligaments (anterior talofibular and calcaneofibular).

of the foot; the PTFL connects to the rear of the talus bone; and the CFL connects to the calcaneus, or heel bone.

### The "Tweaked" Ankle

As many coaches, parents, and players already know from personal experience, the ankle sprain makes up a significant portion (approximately 15%) of the total injuries suffered by soccer athletes at all levels. However, there are many varying degrees of ankle sprains. So, how do you identify an ankle sprain, and how do we treat and prevent it?

Laypeople use all kinds of different terminology to describe an ankle sprain. But whether the ankle is "twisted," "tweaked," "rolled," or "floppy," the ligaments in the foot and ankle have been overstretched, or sprained.

There are several classifications that cover all ligament sprains, and categorize them based on the varying degree of the injury sustained.

### Degrees of Sprains

**First Degree:** Little fibrous tearing of the tissue. Mild swelling and pain, but joint stability is good. Most common, with a fairly short recovery period.

**Second Degree:** Tearing of up to 50%. Moderate pain and associated swelling, along with moderate instability of the joint. Bulbous malleoli (prominent ankle bones made up of tibia and fibula), throbbing and heat at the injury site, and difficulty walking may occur.

**Third Degree:** More than 50% tissue tearing or a complete rupture. The joint is unstable and unable to bear weight, and pain and swelling are severe. This most often occurs in the ATFL or PTFL.

### Mechanism of Injury in Ankle Sprains

Ankle sprains can be caused by some of the simple, daily movements involved with playing soccer. Ankles can be twisted when an athlete comes down from a header and lands on another player's foot. Athletes can turn awkwardly and catch a foot in the turf while pivoting sharply or rotating. Ankles can be rolled from simply running on an uneven surface or falling into a divot, which can forcefully invert the ankle.

The risk involved with any activity is greatest when explosive side-to-side motion is involved. In soccer, athletes perform these kinds of movements all the time, so the opportunity for injury is certainly ever-present throughout the length of the match. Injury risk will increase based on external and environmental factors, such as playing on wet, cold, or hard turf, especially if the athlete is wearing rubber cleats.

### So I've Sprained My Ankle ... Now What?!

Often, at a sanctioned athletic event, there is an onsite certified athletic trainer (ATC) who is overseeing the medical coverage for that event. This professional is capable of identifying and evaluating the extent of injury and defining a plan of care for the athlete. The athlete will often need further medical intervention, such as an x-ray or MRI, but that is up to the evaluating physician to prescribe. These tools help the medical professional see further into any minor complexities associated with the acute injury, which can range from an avulsion, in which the bone on the inside of the ankle pulls away from the ligament, to a complete fracture.

Once the extent of structural damage is established by a physician, it is common to seek out a physical therapist for proper care and treatment of the sprain. The physical therapist is capable of treating ankle sprains of all degrees, including fractures, the reduced or dislocated ankle, and the postoperative ankle.

It is often necessary for the athletic trainer to immobilize immediately and/or put the athlete on crutches, depending on the athlete's gait and ability to bear weight. Immobilization can be done in a walking CAM (controlled ankle motion) boot, a non-weight-bearing (NWB) brace, or a cast applied by a physician. The severity of dysfunction will dictate the length of time allocated for proper healing of the various anatomical structures.

### Treatment of the Acute Ankle Injury

When talking about treatment, it is important to consider the extent of damage, and the amount of healing time associated with the diagnosis of the injured ankle. It is common to develop chronic ankle instability from improper care of and attention to the initial acute ankle sprain. Further damage may even be done to the bone or cartilage of the surrounding joint if a proper treatment protocol is not followed.

As always, RICE! (see chart on page 4) Rest, ice, compression, and elevation will help to limit or decrease the initial inflammatory response. The more swollen the ankle is, the more unstable the ankle is, and the more pain you will feel. The quicker you resolve this response, the more stable the ankle will sit and the quicker you can return to the pitch.

If properly cared for from day one, an athlete with a first-degree sprain can typically be back to full-go within two weeks, assuming there are no lingering issues of soreness or swelling. Second- and third-degree sprains will take much longer to heal, anywhere from one to six months. Injuries with further structural damage to the ligaments and/or tendons will likely need to go through a non-weight-bearing phase and immobilization. This will result in the atrophy of the surrounding musculature; it will get weaker from a lack of use. If an athlete compares the size of the injured foot, calf, and ankle when it comes out of the boot to the uninjured side, he or she will often notice the injured leg is considerably smaller. For this individual, an appropriate treatment plan will include strengthening and restoration of functional movement patterns, which includes exercises to improve balance and proprioception.

## Skeletal Muscle Pump

Swelling in our bodies is sort of a necessary evil. It's our body's way of flooding an injured area with cells that assist in recovery. We need to let the body do its thing, but there are some techniques that can assist the process and limit the amount of time lost from injury.

Always, with initial trauma, our immediate goal is to limit the amount of inflammation that is rushing to the area. Our body is great at healing itself, and it will do just that over a period of time if left to its own devices. However, with less severe sprains and strains, it can be beneficial to activate what's known as our *skeletal muscle pump*. This process activates our lymphatic system, which is connected to our skeletal muscle and is responsible carrying fluid in the body through motion and assists it in picking up excess fluid. As it relates to ankle strains, a gentle flexion and extension of the ankle done in a "pumping" manner can help to increase lymphatic flow and decrease inflammation.

The quicker the initial swelling goes down, the quicker the athlete can advance to the next phase of the treatment protocol. Ideally, the injured ankle (or any injured joint), should be kept above the level of the heart as much as possible so gravity can assist in the process. Lying on the back with the foot propped up (the higher the better), or on the stomach with a bent knee (ankle in the air) are both acceptable.

### The Eight Goals of Rehabilitation

There are eight goals that every physical therapist or athletic trainer will have an athlete accomplish during the rehabilitation of an injury. The completion of these benchmark steps helps to ensure proper recovery and ultimately a return to play.

**Control Pain and Inflammation:** Swelling must be decreased to limit the amount of secondary cell death from the body's natural response to injury. Utilize the RICE protocol (see page 4).

**Restore Range of Motion (ROM):** Increase the amount of motion allowed at a joint that is otherwise limited due to injured tissue or swelling and edema. For example, normal knee ROM is approximately 0° to 135°, and full ROM must be achieved for successful performance. Remember, certain postsurgical guidelines specifically limit ROM for a reason, and certain benchmarks should only be reached at specific times.

**Restore Flexibility:** Most injury prevention protocols include programs to improve extensibility, or a muscle or muscle group's ability to be stretched, as limited extensibility is often partly to blame for the injury itself, and can result in secondary problems.

**Restore Muscular Strength and Endurance:** The health of the muscle is important for good control of an injured limb, especially a lower extremity that must bear weight. Trauma often results in muscular inhibition, or a muscle's inability to fire rly, and must be restored through therapy.

ore Balance and Proprioception: An athlete must have er a limb in an often-unstable environment, as well as have an awareness of a limb or joint's position in space. The athlete must be able to react and respond to an unstable surface while maintaining balance, control, and stability in the injured limb (see Figure 3.2).

**Restore Cardiovascular Endurance:** It is essential for athletes to maintain as much fitness as possible while away from the field. If a return to sport is expected in a short to medium time frame, including low-impact conditioning activities such as stationary biking or swimming with the rehab program is beneficial to deter de-conditioning.

**Return to Functional Training:** To bridge the gap from the table to the field, the rehab program should include functional training activities that mimic on-field agilities and reactions in a controlled environment, such as ladder drills, figure-8 runs, and shuffling and backpedaling (see Figures 3.3–3.5).

**Return to Sport-Specific Training:** The last step prior to a return to practice and game play is to advance to a level of training that involves any and all activities that simulate real-time game situations, but in a controlled environment. For soccer players, this should include soccer positioning drills, shots on goal, and throw-ins.

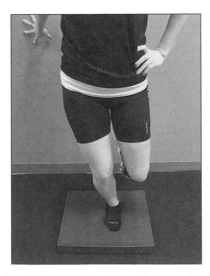

**Figure 3.2** Single leg stance on the Airex Balance Pad: Without a shoe, stand with a slightly bent knee on the Airex Balance Pad for 30 seconds. Repeat three times. The unstable surface activates the proprioceptors in the lower extremity and tests your balance.

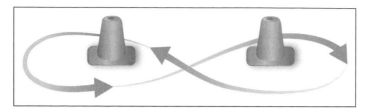

**Figure 3.3** Figure-8 run: Start in the middle of the cones and run in a Figure-8 pattern around the cones, keeping as close to the cones as possible.

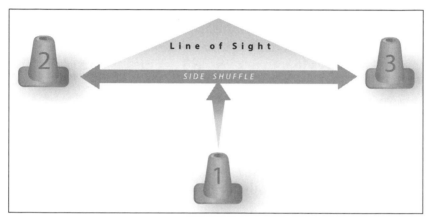

**Figure 3.4** T-test: Start at cone 1. Sprint straight ahead. Side-shuffle to cone 2. Side-shuffle to cone 3. Side-shuffle back to the middle. Backpedal to cone 1.

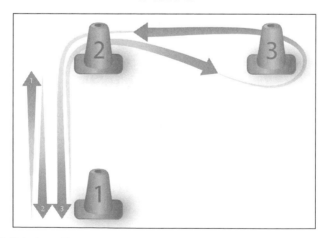

**Figure 3.5** L-test: Start at cone 1. Sprint and touch the line at cone 2. Turn around and sprint back to touch the line at cone 1. Turn around, sprint around cone 2, circle cone 3 in a counter-clockwise direction. Stay to the outside of cone 2 and finish through cone 1.

**Prevention of Ankle Sprains**

Any ATC will tell you that the best way to treat any injury is to avoid it altogether. Many coaches believe ankle bracing and taping can prevent injury by assisting with ankle stability. While it is true the utilization of prophylactic ankle bracing and taping can assist with ankle stability, it is debated whether they can prevent ankle injuries altogether. In some cases, bracing can actually decrease the strength of the surrounding musculature, which may increase the risk of injury while not wearing the brace during participation.

A lower-body strength program that involves both closed kinetic chain (CKC) and open kinetic chain (OKC) exercises, and targets all of the eight benchmark factors listed on pages 40–41 in the treatment section, is considerably more effective than prophylactic bracing and taping. Why wait until there is a problem to fix when we can avoid it altogether with a simple protocol? Of course, we are not claiming that injuries will become nonexistent, but proper strength training can dramatically decrease the risk of injury per athletic exposure.

To prevent re-injury once an athlete returns to play, it is essential to make sure the initial or acute ankle injury is treated and healed appropriately prior to a full return to sport. Following the initial trauma, secondary injuries and sprains happen much more easily and issues can become chronic, so it is important to focus on maintaining strength and flexibility. If you continue to roll on that ankle and have yet to seek out a medical professional, it is time to do so now!

**SYNDESMOTIC OR "HIGH" ANKLE SPRAIN**

While normal ankle sprains occur below the ankle bone when the foot twists forcefully inward, syndesmotic or "high" ankle sprains occur above the ankle bone when the foot twists forcefully inward. The structures most often associated with this injury are the anterior inferior tibiofibular ligament, posterior inferior tibiofibular ligament, and the interosseous membrane. As described earlier, the ankle is in its most stable position when the foot is flexed. However, if the foot is forced into that position, there are structures that can fail and rupture despite being in a position of stability.

**Mechanism of Injury for High Ankle Sprains**

The mechanism of injury for a high ankle sprain is, again, a forceful dorsiflexion and eversion of the ankle; that is, the foot over-flexes upward and the ankle rolls outward. This is often a result of a collision with another player, when the foot is firmly planted into the turf and the opposing player lands on top of the athlete, forcibly separating the bones of the ankle mortise. Pain tends to ride high above the ankle, and really not in the ankle joint itself. This injury is generally less common, but is seen very often in soccer.

High ankle sprains also can occur when a soccer player on the offensive tries to dribble past a defender and loses footing from on top of the ball, causing the forefoot to roll off the ball and catch the ground. Again, the ankle mortise will be forcefully shifted outward, damaging the ligaments that keep it stable. These types of sprains should always to be evaluated by a medical professional.

**Signs and Symptoms of High Ankle Sprains**

Often, a high ankle sprain presents as a dull or sharp pain on the outside of the lower leg along the length of the fibula. This is increased to a much sharper pain with inversion and eversion, especially in a weight-bearing position.

These sprains are generally more difficult to diagnose because swelling is not always as prevalent as it is with a normal ankle sprain. This injury is very often underestimated by coaches, players, and parents. Depending on the extent of tissue damage, this injury can require up to four to six months of recovery. Keep in mind that this time frame does not necessarily include an associated fracture. Due to the location and action required by the ankle, it is difficult to recover in any sort of timely fashion, and we must allow the ligaments sufficient healing time prior to putting them through the stress of rehabilitation.

A true diagnosis of a high ankle sprain can only be made by a physician using an x-ray or MRI. An athletic trainer or physical therapist is certainly capable of coming to the same conclusion through an evaluation that includes a squeeze test of the tibiofibular joint and an eversion stress test, but in order to make a specific diagnosis, the integrity of the ankle mortise must be assessed with more advanced diagnostic tools.

X-ray and MRI can show how far the tibiofibular space has been translated. Essentially, increased tissue damage correlates directly with a widening of the ankle mortise, which can only be seen with advanced imaging. This type of unstable tearing can sometimes lead to extensive long-term treatment, with some sort of surgical procedure to reduce the spacing of the ankle mortise and improve the integrity of the joint.

This type of surgery is not fun. It includes screwing the tibia and fibula together to re-establish the position of the mortise. Rehabilitation with a physical therapist or athletic trainer is crucial, whether or not surgical intervention was necessary, and will be discussed in the following section.

### Treatment of the High Ankle Sprain

A high ankle sprain is treated with the same principles as the lateral ankle sprain. Once again, the extent of tissue damage will dictate the time frame of recovery.

The athlete will typically be placed in a walking boot, immobilizer brace, or hard cast for approximately four to six weeks. It is important to keep the athlete non-weight-bearing to allow for sufficient scarring and tissue healing, in an attempt to regain the integrity of the ankle mortise. Do not be overly aggressive and begin a return-to-play protocol too quickly! Treatment must be conservative to allow the body to heal naturally and reduce the spacing between the bones.

Once cleared to begin a rehab protocol, the initial goal is pain-free weight-bearing activity. Dull aches are common after being immobilized for any amount of time, but if pain is persistent with normal ambulation, progressive resistive exercises (PREs), will be of no benefit. Appropriate steps must be taken in sequence. A foundation of strength through muscle-setting exercises must be established prior to advancing the protocol into closed kinetic chain, balance, and functional strength exercises. Remember, all the muscles surrounding the ankle must be strengthened to give stability to the entire joint (see Figures 3.6–3.8).

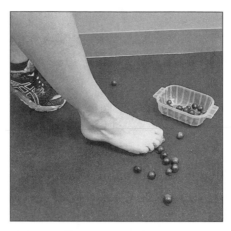

**Figure 3.6** Toe pick-ups: This therapeutic exercise increases Foot and ankle range of motion and strengthens the intrinsic foot musculature. Simply pick up the marble or object with your toes and place in the container.

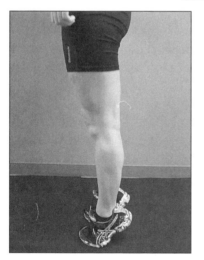 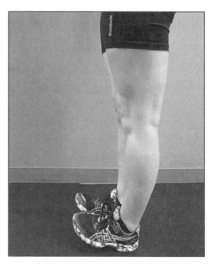

**Figure 3.7** Heel raise: Standing with support, flex the calves and rise up off the heels. Perform three sets of 10 reps.

**Figure 3.8** Toe raise: Standing with support, flex the front of the shin and rise up off the toes. Perform three sets of 10 reps.

## PLANTAR FASCIITIS

Plantar fasciitis can result from either an acute or chronic trauma to the bottom of the foot, and occurs most often in the running athlete. Realize that this injury will keep you out of the game and will not get better with continued running and activity! Treating plantar fasciitis is often difficult for athletic trainers and physical therapists because athletes are unwilling to allow for proper rest and healing. In addition, soccer athletes are often reluctant to use any sort of tape or brace that could alleviate their pain during activity because they fear it will diminish their "touch" or "feel" on the ball.

### Anatomical Makeup

The plantar fascia is the thick band of connective tissue and associated ligaments that runs along the sole of the foot, from the bottom of the heel to the base of the toes. When the plantar fascia becomes inflamed, an athlete will feel pain in the bottom of the foot, most notably in the heel.

To visualize the swelling of the plantar fascia tissue, imagine a sausage in a casing. If the casing is overstuffed, the casing will rupture. Rupturing of the plantar fascia is uncommon, but as with the sausage, there is only so much space available within the fascial sheath, and an increase in swelling with continued activity will cause greater discomfort and disability.

A good way to visualize the action of the plantar fascia is to come back to our rubber band analogy. Envision a proper concave arch running along the bottom of your foot. Now attach several taut rubber bands from the base of your heel to the base of each toe. Got it? Now, take your shoe off and step down a flat surface. What happens to your foot? It splays! As the foot spreads out, the over-taut rubber bands will be stressed even more. The same thing happens to the plantar fascia when it is tight and inflamed. There is not much room for movement.

### Mechanism of Injury for Plantar Fasciitis

There are even some predisposing anatomical conditions that can lead to this pain, including pes planus or "flat feet," and the hyperpronation that often accompanies them (see Figure 3.9).

In addition to these factors of flat feet and poor fitting shoes are the actual training activities. There is not one specific activity that will lead to plantar fasciitis, but it is related to the amount of training and conditioning that an athlete participates in on a weekly basis. This injury will usually happen through continual running, irritating the area under the arch.

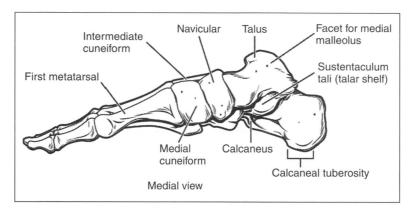

**Figure 3.9** Anatomy: Medial arch of foot.

*Source*: Image reprinted with permission from OpenStax College, *Anatomy & Physiology—Connexions.*

## Signs and Symptoms of Plantar Fasciitis

Most initial complaints about plantar fasciitis pertain to the feeling of the soccer cleat on the foot; athletes will say their shoe is too tight, too flat, or generally uncomfortable.

Essentially, what is being described is an overstretching of the fascial tissue. Most commonly, after being non-weight-bearing for an extended period of time, such as while sitting or sleeping, the fascia has a chance to tighten up. When we stand up and put pressure across this tissue through the splaying of the foot, a sharp pain is noted from the mid-foot to the heel. Pain can be reproduced with forced dorsiflexion and toe extension, occurring simultaneously. This is often done during the evaluation and is a good indicator of this disorder.

The onset of plantar fasciitis can happen acutely with an overextension of the sole on the foot, but is often more consistent with a progressive onset. As is true with any inflammatory process, the increased swelling or edema in the surrounding tissue will cause pain and tightness. This is typically exacerbated following long periods of rest. This is not an injury to which only soccer players are prone; millions of people suffer from plantar fasciitis at some point in their lifetime.

Plantar fasciitis is exacerbated in soccer players because they train in multiple pairs of shoes to accommodate the frequent change in training surfaces. By limiting those variables, along with training hours, we can begin to scale back some of the damage already done. Long-standing cases of plantar fasciitis can sometimes cause a degenerative change in the tissue, and lead to more inflammation that can potentially cause fibrous tearing of the connective tissue of both the surrounding ligaments and tendons.

The diagnosis of plantar fasciitis is made by a medical professional through examination of the involved tissues. To properly evaluate the integrity of the medial longitudinal arch (the primary arch along the inside of your foot running from heel to toe), the patient should be barefoot, and observed in both non-weight-bearing and full weight-bearing positions. Further evaluation may involve advanced imaging in order to quantify the inflammation in the fascial tissue.

**Treatment of Plantar Fasciitis**

The simplistic approach to treatment of plantar fasciitis is to decrease the inflammation. This can be done through prescription anti-inflammatory drugs, but keep in mind there will be more long-term improvement if the actual cause of the inflammation is addressed! If inflammation is severe, it may be in the best interest of the athlete to spend some time in a boot. Of course, the RICE protocol still applies (see chart on page 4). Ice is most effectively applied to this area by giving the athlete a frozen bottle of water to roll along the sole of the foot while in a seated position.

Once the athlete becomes pain-free, flexibility of the connective tissue must be restored. The goal is to stretch the fascia, along with the heel cord and lower-leg, into a dorsiflexion. This will give elasticity to the entire structure, and work on some of the predisposing factors.

In physical therapy and athletic training, we will use electric modalities, massage, and stretching techniques to loosen the tissue and decrease inflammation. Simple exercises will also be used to strengthen the bottom of the foot, advancing to more weight-bearing or closed kinetic chain strengthening exercises as the athlete progresses. Then, balance and proprioceptive components will be added before moving into functional and sport-specific training. Balance exercises teach the body to react appropriately to sudden changes in the environment. Proprioceptive exercises increase the body's awareness of a joint or limb's position in space and time. The same exercises can be done to improve both balance and proprioception, but they will be done with the eyes open to work on balance and the eyes closed to work on proprioception.

There is no quick fix for plantar fasciitis. It requires a time-consuming rehabilitation process. If the athlete does not respond to therapy, physicians may consider a corticosteroid injection to assist in the healing process. If still no progress is made, there are many different surgical techniques that can be used to release the tension in the plantar fascia.

### Prevention of Plantar Fasciitis

As with every other part of the body, a proper warm-up is key. Athletes are always very concerned about loosening up their hamstrings and quadriceps, but they often forget that running athletes need their feet! The tissue at the sole of the foot needs to be kept elastic, as inelasticity leads to dysfunction. One good stretch for the plantar fascia entails wedging the foot against a wall, with the toes flexed back toward the ankle.

Inserts, both store-bought and custom-made, may be added to footwear to provide medial arch stability and help with the positioning of the foot within the shoe. A medical professional can aide in the selection of such products.

For those with recurrent plantar fasciitis, night splints can be beneficial to help keep the fascia in a stretched position during sleep.

An athletic trainer or physical therapist can also use a technique called low-dye arch taping to support the plantar fascia in a way that mimics an orthotic or over-the-counter shoe insert.

### METATARSALGIA

Metatarsalgia is a tough word to say, but it simply refers to that nagging pain at the ball of your foot. It is most often caused by … surprise … inflammation! Running and jumping athletes can develop metatarsalgia simply through overuse, but the tight fit of the shoes worn by the majority of soccer players can hasten its onset. Sometimes, shoes can actually be so tight as to cause an inflammatory process, with symptoms that include sharp, achy, burning pain in the ball of the foot, directly behind the toes.

**Anatomical Makeup**

The metatarsals are the five bones that run from your mid-foot to each toe. Anatomically, the first and second metatarsals, those that correspond to the big toe and second toe, are shorter and thicker than the other three, and similar in size. During push-off, body weight is transferred to the heads of the metatarsals, and the first two absorb the majority of the force.

**Mechanism of Injury for Metatarsalgia**

Metatarsalgia can be an acute injury resulting from a rapid increase in running or jumping activity, or a chronic injury that develops over a long period of running and jumping.

Deviations in gait patterns and anatomical discrepancies can predispose an individual to this injury. If an athlete is coming back from another injury and is favoring one side, his or her gait may be altered. A bruise to another part of the foot can change the way an athlete strides and places his or her foot down. The ill-effects of these deviations are compounded with repetitive pounding, especially in footwear that doesn't fit properly or is worn out. Other factors, such as being overweight, wearing high-heeled shoes, or having extremely high arches can contribute to metatarsalgia.

**Signs and Symptoms of Metatarsalgia**

Pain is most often felt at the base of toes two through four, moving from the big toe to the pinky toe. Pain increases with standing, walking, and running, but can improve when the shoe is taken off. Some athletes describe this pain as similar to the feeling of having a rock in their shoe. Basically the part of the foot that propels the body forward during push-off in walking and running becomes inflamed, irritated, and very sensitive.

**Treatment of Metatarsalgia**

Treatment for metatarsalgia targets the inflammation around the metatarsal heads. The RICE protocol (see chart on page 4), electric stimulation, ultrasound, and laser therapy can assist in the reduction of inflammation. As the body reabsorbs excess inflammation, and the antagonist is removed, pain will begin to subside. If symptoms persist, the physical therapist or athletic trainer may elect to have the athlete rest in a CAM boot, which will take the pressure off the metatarsal heads at the ball of the foot.

A physician may also elect to prescribe an anti-inflammatory drug to decrease the inflammation and pain. Possibilities include ibuprofen, acetaminophen, and naproxen, which are all nonsteroidal anti-inflammatory drugs, or NSAIDs.

### Prevention of Metatarsalgia

One simple way to prevent metatarsalgia is to wear proper-fitting shoes. When recovering from metatarsalgia, it is important to not come back too soon, and to utilize a clear, logical, and gradual progression back into activity. To prevent recurring pain, metatarsal pads, which can be found in most pharmacies, can also be used. These pads help to distribute the weight and force of the foot away from the metatarsal heads, and cut down on the pressure occurring directly at the site of inflammation.

### LISFRANC FRACTURE

Lisfranc fractures, named for the French surgeon who first described them in the early 1800s, occur in the mid-foot, affecting the five bones that make up this portion of the foot (see Figure 3.10). The importance of the mid-foot to a soccer player cannot be overstated. It allows for proper distribution of ground forces from the ball of the foot to the ankle, and ultimately to the rest of the body.

### Anatomical Makeup

The foot, like the wrist, has many small bones with musculotendinous attachments that allow for greater dexterity and flexibility and provide improved motion on uneven surfaces. The Lisfranc joint complex includes the bones, tendons, and ligaments that connect the mid-foot to the forefoot, and forms the arch at the top of the foot. Ligaments and tendons in this area can be sprained, and the bones can be fractured.

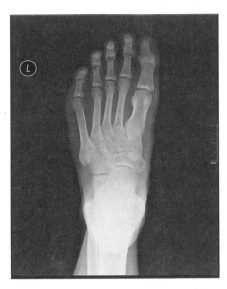

**Figure 3.10** Anatomy: Lisfranc bones of the mid-foot.

The bones of the mid-foot have articulations with all five metatarsals. These bones are the three cuneiforms, the cuboid, and the navicular.

**Mechanism of Injury for a Lisfranc Fracture**

Direct Lisfranc injuries are the result of a trauma. They are often seen in soccer players when the athlete's foot is plantarflexed, or pointed down, and another player steps on or tackles them, causing a shift in their bones. As described above, this can result in either a sprain or a fracture.

Indirect Lisfranc injuries are caused when a sudden rotational force is applied to the mid-foot, whether the force is the result of contact or not. Commonly, a deformity can be seen in the foot. If not as obvious, an x-ray or CT scan should be used to look for a gap between the base of the first and second metatarsals to confirm the diagnosis.

**Classifications of Lisfranc Fractures**

**Homolateral**: This describes a displacement of all bones in the same direction.

**Isolated**: This describes a deviation of one or two bones in the same direction.

**Divergent**: This describes the displacement of the metatarsals in varying directions

### Treatment of Lisfranc Fractures

If surgery is elected, a physician will reduce the dislocation, and may elect to pin the fracture site with an open-reduction internal fixation, or ORIF. This includes a combination of screws and wires to keep the bones and joints intact.

Recovery will include a non-weight-bearing period or a period of partial weight-bearing in a CAM walking boot. This will provide for adequate time to allow the bone to heal. Typically, six to eight weeks are required to allow the bone to set. Around 10 to 12 weeks postsurgery, the physician will remove the screws and wiring. The athlete can then progress to weight-bearing activity, strength and balance exercises, and return-to-play activities.

It is important for the soccer athlete to recognize that recovery will include soreness in the mid-foot, sometimes for upwards of a year, through rehab, running, and playing.

Nonsurgical treatment of a Lisfranc fracture is very similar to surgical rehab. Adequate time must be allowed for bone healing, either non-weight-bearing on crutches or partial weight-bearing in a boot. Then, the athlete can commence with a logical progression into weight-bearing activity, including ROM, flexibility, strength, balance and proprioceptive exercises, functional, and eventually sport-specific conditioning.

### JONES FRACTURES

A Jones fracture refers specifically to a crack at the base of the fifth metatarsal bone in the foot, which leads to the pinky toe, most commonly in the midportion of the foot (see Figure 3.11). It is named for the British surgeon, Sir Robert Jones, who first described it in the early 1900s, after suffering the injury himself while dancing. Pain, swelling, and difficulty walking are common, but still, most athletes don't realize they have a fracture. The only way to obtain a true diagnosis is through x-ray or CT scan.

### Mechanism of Injury for Jones Fractures

Jones fractures most often occur without significant impact or trauma and can happen simply as a result of wearing poor-fitting shoes. If the shoe is too tight around the mid-foot, it can put too much stress on the base of the fifth metatarsal. Jones fractures can also be the result of overuse. No matter the cause, Jones fractures need to be treated by a physician.

### Treatment of Jones Fractures

If there is any spacing within the bone, surgery is required to screw the bone back together. Recovery will include a non-weight-bearing period or a period of partial weight-bearing in a CAM walking boot. This will provide for adequate time to allow the bone to heal. Typically, six to eight weeks are required to allow the bone to set. Around 10 to 12 weeks postsurgery, the physician will remove the screws and wiring. The athlete can

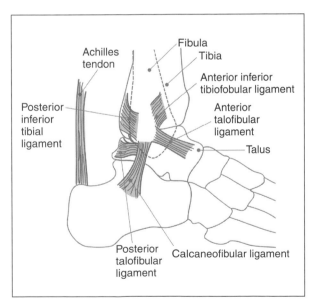

**Figure 3.11** Anatomy: Lateral view of ankle bones.

*Source*: Image courtesy of the National Institute of Arthritis and Musculoskeletal and Skin Diseases.

then progress to weight-bearing activity, strength and balance exercises, and return-to-play activities. There is an outstanding success rate associated with this surgery.

If the Jones fracture is nondisplaced, treatment can be done nonsurgically, with a simple splint or walking boot. As with the Lisfranc fracture, nonsurgical recovery is very similar to that of surgical rehab. Adequate time must be allowed for bone healing, either non-weight-bearing on crutches or partial weight-bearing in a boot. Then the athlete can commence with a logical progression into weight-bearing activity, including ROM, flexibility, strength, balance and proprioceptive exercises, functional, and eventually sport-specific conditioning.

Nonsurgically treated Jones fractures have a very high nonunion rate, which means the bone will not fuse back together. This leads to chronic pain and an inability to perform. Most surgeons or podiatrists will therefore recommend surgery.

# CHAPTER FOUR

# KNEE INJURIES

Some of the most common injuries we see on the soccer field occur in the knee. The knee is one of the most complex joints in the body. It is a hinge joint that allow for minimal rotational translation—that is, side-to-side movement—and acts as a shock absorber for most athletic activities. The knee joins the distal femur, or thighbone, to the proximal tibia, or shinbone. The patella, or kneecap, sits in the concave area at the bottom of the femur known as the trochlear groove (see Figure 4.1).

The knee is the primary shock absorber for the lower body during the running, jumping, cutting, and kicking that happens in soccer. Just like the shock absorbers on a car, the knee joint is subjected to a lot of wear over the length of an athletic career. Of course, the soccer athlete places great demands on the lower body, and will see the majority of injuries in the lower extremities.

There are a number of structures surrounding the knee that support and stabilize the joint. Unlike the ankle, where the bony makeup helps to support the joint in dorsiflexion, the bony makeup of the knee doesn't do much to support its

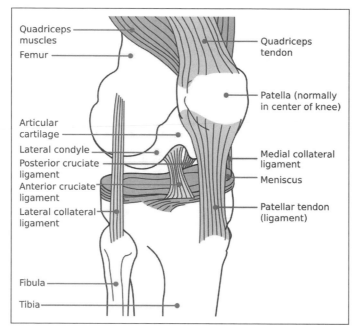

**Figure 4.1**  Anatomy: Anterior view of knee bones.
*Source*: Illustration by Oona Räisänen (MySid).

structural integrity. Instead, the knee has muscles, tendons, ligaments, and cartilage that maintain its stability. Muscularly, the knee is supported by the quadriceps, hamstrings, and calf, specifically the gastrocnemius. The four main ligaments surrounding the knee are the cruciates (anterior and posterior) and collaterals (medial and lateral). The medial and lateral menisci are cartilaginous structures that cushion the knee and balance weight across the joint.

## MEDIAL COLLATERAL LIGAMENT (MCL) INJURIES

The medial collateral ligament (MCL) is located on the medial, or inner, side of the knee, originating at the distal femur and inserting deep into the medial meniscus at the proximal tibia. It is a thick, fibrous band of tissue that is taut when the knee is extended or straightened, and loses internal tension when the knee is flexed or bent. It is important to keep this in mind when considering mechanisms for spraining this structure.

The primary mechanism of injury comes from a strong vagus force (see Figure 4.2), which must be generated externally. A valgus force is a lateral force—that is, from the outside to the inside—that tries to force the knee beyond its normal range of motion. This often happens with either a 50/50 ball, where two players attempt to strike the ball simultaneously, or another player falling onto the outside of the athlete's knee with their foot firmly planted in the ground.

As with all ligaments, there are three grades of ligament damage, ranging in severity.

**GRADE 1:** Few fibers are damaged. There are minor tears and some swelling. More of an overstretching than a tear.

**GRADE 2:** There is more extensive fibrous damage but a good portion of the ligament is still intact.

**GRADE 3:** Complete, full-thickness rupture of the ligament.

Symptoms of an MCL sprain tear will be an immediate onset of swelling, pain, stiffness, point tenderness over the medial joint

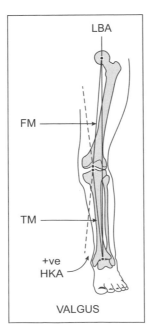

**Figure 4.2** Valgus force at the knee: An external force that crosses the knee from the lateral side to the medial side.

line, and possibly a feeling of instability within the knee joint when walking.

It is up to the medical professional to get a full medical history, detailing exactly what happened to cause the injury, before making a diagnosis. The angle at which force was applied to the knee during injury is important. An experienced athletic trainer will be able to diagnose an MCL sprain to a degree of about 85% certainty based on the description provided by the athlete. Based on the level of discomfort and disability, most sprains fall somewhere in the range between grades 1 and 2. However, if the athlete describes hearing or feeling a "pop" to the inside of the knee, it may be warranted to look further via x-ray or MRI to more accurately assess the level of ligament damage. When a grade 3 tear is suffered, the force of the injury is often such that other structures, such as the medial meniscus or anterior cruciate ligament (ACL), could also be affected.

## Treatment of MCL Injuries

A grade 1 MCL sprain is often referred to as "the 21-day injury." Within 21 days, the athlete should be able to recover and be full-go for a return to sport. However, early intervention is critical to maintaining this time frame. With most grade 1 and grade 2 MCL sprains, it is important to treat with the RICE protocol, and physician-prescribed NSAIDs may further help to decrease inflammation in and around the knee.

When returning to play, it may be helpful to use a double-hinge knee brace to help protect the MCL (see Figure 4.3).

A grade 2 sprain has more structural damage than a grade 1 sprain and therefore requires a longer recovery period. As stated over and over again in this book, if the athlete is progressed too quickly the injury will not heal and the pain and discomfort will continue as the rehabilitation process is dragged out. It is important for the athlete to communicate with the sports medicine staff as to the level of pain or any feelings of instability. If treated appropriately, the athlete can expect a six to eight week rehabilitation process prior to setting foot into a game situation.

When returning to play after a grade 2 MCL strain, most athletes will describe a vibratory sensation in their knee if returning too soon. However, some pain is normal and usually goes

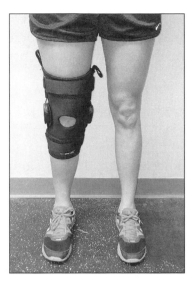

**Figure 4.3** Double-hinge knee brace: Stabilizes and supports side-to-side motion in the knee

away within 7 to 10 days, as long as the athlete continues with a strength and stability program.

If the athlete suffers a grade 3 strain, it will be treated very conservatively. The same benchmarks exist, but with a longer time frame allotted for the early phases of RICE, nonsteroidal anti-inflammatory drug, and possible immobilization. The time-line may also be altered based on the athlete's degree of function. It is up to the orthopedic surgeon to determine if surgical inter-vention is warranted. But regardless of the treatment decided upon, the protocol established by the medical professional will be very similar in all cases.

As always, refer to the eight goals of rehab (see pags 40–41) when treating this injury.

### Prevention of MCL Injuries

MCL injuries can be prevented to a certain extent by following a good lower-extremity strengthening program that targets the quad-riceps and hamstrings and will assist the ligaments in maintaining the stability of the knee. Also, warming up appropriately can help prepare the knee joint and the surrounding structures for action; warm tissue is much less susceptible to injury than cold tissue.

However, soccer is a contact sport, and despite all precau-tions, injuries happen. Little can be done to completely prevent an MCL injury, though if a soccer athlete is returning to play from a prior MCL sprain, a double-hinge knee brace can help prevent re-injury by assisting the structures that support the MCL.

### LATERAL COLLATERAL LIGAMENT SPRAINS AND TEARS

The lateral collateral ligament, or LCL, plays a smaller role than that of the MCL in knee stability. It runs along the outside of the knee, starting at the distal lateral femur and ending at the proximal lateral tibia. The position of the LCL over the lateral joint line somewhat protects it from injury, because it is difficult for athletes to create enough varus force to cause injury, either on their own or with contact with others (see Figure 4.4).

The same three grades for ligament damage classification listed above exist with the LCL sprain. However, the mechanism of injury is different. LCL injuries may result from a collision during a 50/50 ball, but more often they are seen with collisions or contact that create a strong varus force. Varus stress is a medial

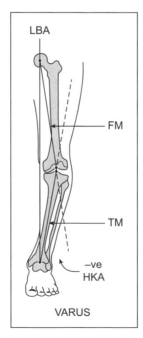

**Figure 4.4** Varus force at the knee: An external force that crosses the knee from the medial side to the lateral side.

force that travels from the inside to the outside of the knee and tries to force the joint beyond it's normal range of motion.

As discussed with the MCL, rehabilitative guidelines and prevention guidelines for the LCL are similar. MCL injuries are more common among soccer athletes, and more games are lost to MCL injuries than to LCL injuries.

## ACL INJURIES

Contained deep inside your knee joint are two cruciate ligments, so defined because they cross over each other in a pattern that looks like the letter "X." These cruciate ligaments work to resist torsional, or twisting, and translational, or side-to-side, forces of the tibia on the femur. The posterior cruciate ligament, or PCL, runs from the posterior tibia to the medial femoral condyle, resisting posterior tibial translation and external tibial rotation on the femur. The ACL runs from the posterior wall of the lateral femoral condyle to the anterior tibia, resisting anterior translation of the tibia on the femur and internal tibial rotation. More simply put, the PCL resists forces that would push the tibia back in relation to the femur, while the ACL resists forces that would push it forward.

The reason I included such a long-winded explanation here is to detail the action that these ligaments provide in knee stabilization. These ligaments are very thick bands of fibrous tissue that provide much stability around a knee that has little else keeping it intact. They are especially important to athletes who play the dynamic sport of soccer. Injury to these structures, especially the ACL, will cause a certain level of instability in the knee. Athletes will often describe a feeling of "buckling" when walking. It is important to note that the unstable knee is at risk for developing secondary injuries to other supporting structures, especially if athletic participation is continued.

### Mechanism of Injury for ACL Injuries

There are many ways an athlete can tear the ACL, but all the mechanisms of injury fall under two categories: contact and noncontact. (Contact is generally used in reference to contact with an opposing athlete.)

A contact injury to the ACL describes a mechanism of injury in which the knee is subjected to a sudden valgus force through contact with another athlete. The force is great enough to open the knee joint to such an extent that the ACL tears. Often, we see this mechanism with an offensive player being "rolled up on" by another player. This type of injury can range in severity based on the tissues that are damaged. In the worst case, an athlete will suffer "the unhappy triad," which refers to a rupture of the MCL, medial meniscus, and ACL. Surgical repair is required in such an instance.

Noncontact injuries to the ACL are most often caused by a sudden twist or forceful contraction of the quadriceps with the foot planted and the knee in a valgus, or knock-kneed, position. Often, a sudden stop and change of direction where the athlete firmly plants their foot in the turf is enough to stress this ligament beyond its tensile strength. Keep in mind, the tensile strength of this ligament is tremendous, but everything has its breaking point.

The ACL can also suffer a noncontact trauma through a forceful contraction of the quadriceps, which can pull the tibia forward on the femur with enough force to tear the ACL. This happens most often when an athlete's foot is planted on the ground and he or she then makes an awkward twisting or cutting movement.

### Signs and Symptoms of ACL Injuries

If the athletic trainer is in a good position to see the mechanism of injury clearly, then 85% of the evaluation is already done. The job at this point is to calm the athlete and collect information. After determining that an ambulance is not necessary, it is appropriate to palpate and test the knee's range of motion, possibly including a Lachmann or anterior drawer test, which manually stresses the ACL to check for instability. It is best to do this test on the field right after the injury occurs because the muscles surrounding the knee will tighten up to protect the injury site. Once this muscle-guarding response happens, it is more difficult for a medical professional to diagnose an ACL tear with a physical examination.

Symptoms often described by the athlete include the feeling of a sometimes audible "pop," with immediate swelling, a feeling of instability, and difficulty bearing weight. Because this injury has become so prevalent in our athletic culture, everyone tends to fear the worst. Fortunately, protocols for identifying, correcting, and restoring the athlete back to prior function are on the cutting edge. The time between initial injury and full return to play has been cut down to less than one year! This, of course, assumes there has been early intervention, and no difficulties have arisen throughout the course of rehabilitation.

## Treatment of ACL Injuries

When a suspected ACL tear is sustained on-field, it is important for the athlete to have the knee immobilized, keep the limb non-weight-bearing and, if possible, RICE to limit the pain and inflammation. After the athletic trainer completes the on-field assessment, the athlete's status will be determined and a plan of care for further evaluation by a physician will be recommended.

Depending on circumstances (the athlete's level of pain and mobility, accessibility of care, etc.), it is acceptable to wait a day or two to see an orthopedist. This is not normally an injury that requires immediate medical attention, but the athlete should contact a local orthopedic surgeon right away in order to schedule an appointment.

Some parents prefer the peace of mind afforded by taking their child to the emergency room and getting a more immediate diagnosis. But do keep in mind that many outpatient medical centers (not hospital ERs) provide the luxury of being fast-tracked in order to help speed up the process of having an orthopedic evaluation and of scheduling further diagnostic testing. If the physician confirms the likelihood of knee injury, conclusive evidence can be seen through an MRI in order to properly define the variance of the tear, and the athlete can immediately move forward to a preoperative rehabilitation protocol to prep for surgery.

## Surgical Repair of the ACL

ACL injuries are surgically corrected about 90% of the time. Presurgical rehabilitation has been proven to improve postsurgical outcomes, and is necessary to reduce the initial inflammatory response from trauma. Along with controlling the pain and inflammation posttrauma, the goal of the physical therapist is to restore basic range of motion from 0° to 110° of flexion. Additionally, muscle activation via muscle-setting exercises helps to restore normal neurological muscle-firing patterns.

Posttrauma, muscles can shut down in a neurological response known as muscular inhibition. If the muscles cannot be fully activated, the limitation can negatively affect rehabilitation.

Most orthopedists will perform surgery 14 to 21 days posttrauma, to allow the body's initial inflammatory response to calm down prior to introducing the entirely new trauma that is surgical repair.

When performing ACL surgery, doctors want to replace the torn ACL with a ligament that is of similar thickness and tensile strength. Options include the autograft, which is tissue taken from the patient's own body, or the allograft, which is tissue taken from a cadaver.

The two most commonly used autograft tendons are the patellar tendon and the hamstring tendon. Because the patellar tendon has bony insertions at either end (it attaches to the patella and tibia), this graft is referred to as a "bone-tendon-bone (BTB) graft. The bone on either end is removed and the tendon is reinserted into tunnels in the femur and tibia. Only the middle third of the patellar tendon is used, leaving the outer portions of the tendon intact to allow for proper functioning of the quadriceps.

Sometimes, in running athletes, there can be some postsurgical anterior knee pain at the site of excision. This area must be given time to heal, and must be considered during the treatment protocol. Adequate recovery time will allow the new implant to heal into the bone. The body will accept it, and the treatment protocol can be progressed.

BTB grafts were first used in the 1980s, when they were considered the gold standard for ACL repair. While they do heal very well and are still considered very reliable, there are now other techniques available.

The hamstring tendon is another autograft that has similar tensile strength to the ACL and yields high rates of success. This is similar to the BTB graft in every respect, except for the obvious location of excision, and the fact that it is all tendon, rather than beginning and ending with bone. Using a graft from the hamstring tendon will not affect hamstring strength in the long term.

The most commonly used allograft, or cadaver tissue, is the Achilles tendon, which is re-formed in the shape of the ACL. It is very strong and is often used based on availability.

However, because cadaver tissue is a foreign substance that will be placed in the patient's body, there is a small risk that the graft will not "take," and can be rejected by the body.

All of these grafts are inserted into the femur and tibia, through tunnels that are drilled into the joint, and anchored into place. It generally takes six to eight weeks for the graft to heal into the bone. During this time the graft needs to be protected, and not overstretched or damaged, so stability can be restored to the knee.

It is the general consensus that anyone competing in athletics or who will continue to be physically active throughout their lives needs to have surgery. It is entirely up to the orthopedist and the patient to make this decision. The risk often associated with not surgically repairing this ligament is that of a secondary arthritic condition of the joint cartilage between the femur and tibia.

### Preoperative Care

As stated above, preoperative care is primarily to reduce inflammation, regain some range of motion (see Figure 4.5), and recruit normal neuromuscular control. It is important for the physical therapist to take into account any secondary injuries that might have been sustained, whether to the meniscus or MCL, because they will often cause more pain at certain ranges of motion.

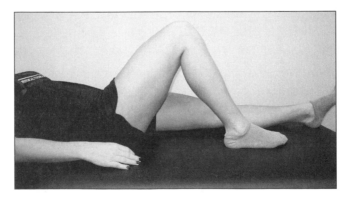

**Figure 4.5** Heel slides: While lying in a supine position with the legs straight out, bend at the knee and slide the heel toward the buttock. Perform 15 repetitions with a three-second pause at the top of each rep.

## Postoperative Care

Most orthopedists are postoperatively aggressive with the ACL. Usually, the athlete will be back in rehab with a physical therapist within 1 to 10 days of the surgery. Although it may seem like a long road ahead for the athlete, the process can be broken down into stages so as not to overwhelm the athlete with time lines. In the early stages, I tell athletes to look at their rehab as three separate eight-week intervals. Keep in mind that although treatment plans will be similar, each orthopedic surgeon has his or her own postsurgical protocol. This often depends on the individual athlete and what exactly was repaired or corrected during surgery.

**Phase I (Weeks 1 to 8):** The most important thing during this stage is to protect the new graft! The new graft must heal into the bone, and needs to be given a chance to scar down into place to restore stability in the knee. Over the course of the first eight weeks, the following should be achieved:

- Decrease pain and inflammation
- Increase ROM from 0° to 90°
- Good vastus medialis oblique (VMO), or quad, contraction
- Manage scarring and incisions
- Progress to full weight-bearing
- Achieve a normal gait pattern

**Phase II (Weeks 9 to 16):** At this point, the graft has had a good chance to heal into the bone. During this eight-week period, the objective is to return joint integrity and strength, using both open and closed kinetic chain exercises. The following should be addressed:

- Working on strength of hip, foot, and ankle.
- Begin leg press
- Functional squats
- Leg curl, leg extension

**Phase III (Weeks 17 to full return to play):** Every athlete enjoys this part of rehab, as they begin to see the light at the end of the tunnel and can begin to return to a higher level of activity. This period should include the following:

- Running
- Directional running

- Lateral motions
- Diagonal motions
- Low-level plyometrics
- Proprioceptive and balance exercises

During these eight weeks, the athlete can also begin sport-specific activity. With the physician's permission, the athlete can begin a return to sport plan, but only while realizing that he or she has not played a soccer game in 6 months and the return to play must be done gradually; no one wants to ruin 6 to 12 months of rehab by rushing back onto the field.

### Predisposing Factors for ACL Injuries

The incidence of ACL tears has been found to be higher in specific populations that have mechanical and physiological factors predisposing them to ACL injury. Listed below are some of these predispositions. Later, we will discuss ways to correct, and to a certain extent, prevent, some of these predispositions. Ultimately, there are certain risks inherent to athletics, and athletes that have any of these factors must determine for themselves whether or not they feel participation is worth the risk.

#### *Q-angle*

It is well documented that females are at a higher risk of ACL tears than males. Research has concluded that the quadriceps angle, or Q-angle, is generally larger in females than males due to a wider pelvis (see Figure 4.6). The Q-angle is defined as the angle at which the femur, or thigh bone, meets the tibia, or shinbone. The Q-angle is calculated by measuring the angle between two lines; one from the anterior superior iliac spine (ASIS) of the pelvis to the middle of the patella, and the other from the middle of the patella to the tibial tubercle, which is the bump just below the knee. As you can see represented in Figure 4.6, a larger Q-angle indicates a greater valgus force at the knee, which puts the ACL under a higher amount of stress.

#### *Hormonal Variance*

The hormonal variance between males and females has also been researched as a possible cause for a higher predisposition toward ACL injuries. Specifically in females during menstruation, higher

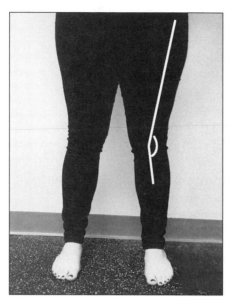

**Figure 4.6** Q-angle: The quadriceps angle is the angle between two intersecting lines; the first from the anterior superior iliac spine, (ASIS) to the middle of the patella, and the second from the tibial tubercle to the middle of the patella.

levels of estrogen and progesterone are recorded and may lead to increased laxity in ligaments throughout the body. Studies have shown that this is a definite possibility, although only significant if combined with other predisposing factors.

### *Muscular Imbalances*

Muscular imbalances between the quadriceps and hamstrings can lead to a higher risk of ACL injury. An overdeveloped quadriceps muscle group can lead to greater anterior translation of the tibia on the femur. This is especially true during high-velocity athletics where a sharp deceleration can cause a strong quadriceps contraction. Proper hamstring strength will assist in pulling back posteriorly on the tibia.

### A Brief Discussion of Partial ACL Tears

Studies have shown that surgery is recommended to repair any fibrous tearing of the ACL greater than 50% of full thickness. Of course, there are many factors that may contribute to this decision. How deep is the athlete into the season? Is the athlete returning next season? What is the athlete's current functional level? What functionality does the athlete's sport demand?

All of these things must be considered in an open dialog between the athlete and the physician. The athlete must be realistic as to the expectation of playing at a higher level, and the athlete's safety must be taken into account. Perhaps the most important question to ask is this: What are the long-term effects of living with a partially torn ACL?

### Prevention of ACL Injuries

As the incidence of ACL injuries has increased in recent years, programs have been developed to target the prevention of knee injuries, specifically the ACL. Evidence-based research has shown, especially with the female athlete, that with proper conditioning, we can truly decrease the incidence of ACL tears.

These programs are simple and can be applied to any athlete at all ages and levels of competition. Essentially, the programs teach the athlete to have proper body mechanics in the actions of jumping, landing, and rotating. While these are natural movements, a large portion of the population does not move through them properly. By retraining the body's movement patterns and decreasing vulnerabilities, injury risk can be limited to a certain extent.

Ultimately, whatever route you choose will give you the ability to decrease your risk for ACL instability. I'm of the mindset that if you can reduce the potential loss of a season by taking an extra 15 minutes before practice to properly warm-up, why wouldn't you? My LESS program is based on the most current research available. While it is good for strengthening the entire lower extremity group, it was specifically designed for the prevention of ACL injuries. The JAG Physical Therapy LESS Program is outlined on pages 171–184.

### MENISCUS INJURIES

The menisci act as shock absorbers within the knee joint and provide lubrication during flexion and extension of the knee. They are rubbery, cartilaginous cushions that attach to the proximal tibial plateau, which is the area within the joint that is in contact with the femur, or thigh bone. The meniscus is made up of two portions that are slightly different in shape. The medial meniscus is a C-shaped crescent, whereas the lateral meniscus is more of a closed O-shape.

Meniscus tears are very common in the soccer athlete, and sometimes require surgical intervention. Proper identification of this injury can be made through evaluation, but because the knee is a very complex joint, diagnosis can prove difficult. Most athletes will describe a catching or clicking when they bend their knee, often with intense pain. However, most athletes' knees, ankles, and hips will catch, click, and pop every day, without much cause for concern. It is up to the professional to determine what is normal and what is not.

## Mechanism of Injury to the Meniscus

Different mechanisms can cause meniscus tears, but they are most commonly sustained during a deep squat with a twist. With increased dynamics in this position, there is a greater risk for insult to the cartilage between the bones.

### Biomechanics of the Deep Squat

The meniscus is primarily in contact with the femur, and specifically the femoral condyles, which are the two projections at the bottom of the femur. The condyles are thicker anteriorly than they are posteriorly. Biomechanically, when the knee is in full extension, the surface area in contact with the meniscus is at its greatest. Greater contact area means greater distribution of forces through the menisci.

Alternatively, when the knee is in a position of *greater* than 90° of flexion, as is always seen in the deep squat, the contact area of the femoral condyles with the menisci is at its lowest. Biomechanically, less surface area in contact with the meniscus will increase the amount of force transmitted through those two points of contact.

Remember, the menisci are our primary shock absorbers in the knee. Improper wearing of these structures will lead to degenerative changes resulting in pain and discomfort. While deep squats can cause degeneration, this position is often unavoidable in both athletics and everyday life, so it can be beneficial to train the body to be comfortable in that position, with reason and without excess. If it hurts, don't do it.

### Signs and Symptoms of Meniscus Injuries

There are several general classifications of meniscus tears, named for the way they look on radiographs: longitudinal, bucket handle, parrot beak, or mixed bundle, which is a mixture of all three. Meniscus tears present in three different ways, depending on the onset of symptoms.

### *Acute*

If an athlete feels a "pop" during a deep knee bend, he or she likely has an acute meniscus tear. Athletic trainers will likely observe swelling, joint stiffness, and an associated locking of the knee in a flexed position. The locking is often a result of actually having a flap of the torn meniscus caught in the joint, causing extreme pain at certain ranges of motion.

### *Subacute*

Subacute meniscus tears cause pain without affecting the functionality of the knee. They generally hurt less than acute tears; however, over time, symptoms may increase and can result in long-term pain and degeneration. If not treated appropriately, the persistent inflammation and lack of a complete meniscus can cause an instability of the joint, resulting in further injury.

### *Chronic*

Most older soccer athletes have some level of degeneration in their meniscus, based on a wearing or thinning over time from years of abuse. The level of pain varies with the individual. Depending on the circumstances, this player may want to consider making the transition to coaching! If degeneration is very advanced, a partial or total knee replacement may be necessary.

### Treatment of Meniscus Injuries

Depending on the onset of symptoms (acute, subacute, or chronic), it is advised to RICE! Based on pain level and functionality, crutches may be necessary to make the athlete non-weight-bearing, and NSAIDs can be used to decrease inflammation and pain.

To properly care for and treat the meniscus, it is important to have an understanding of the blood supply to the different areas of the menisci. The outside one-third of the meniscus has a rich blood supply, and tears in this area, while often repaired with surgery, can sometimes heal on their own. In contrast, the inner two-thirds of the meniscus lacks blood supply, which means tears in this area cannot heal.

The location of a meniscus tear will often dictate whether or not surgery is required. If a tear occurs in an area where there is good blood supply, the body will be able to heal naturally. Without good blood supply, the tissue will simply float in the joint and continue to cause pain and discomfort. Because the body cannot heal tears in these locations, suturing the torn tissue will not provide any benefit. In this instance, it is better to just remove the torn or frayed cartilage altogether.

Surgically, meniscus tears can usually be fixed arthroscopically, with minimal invasiveness. As mentioned earlier, surgical technique to either repair or remove a section of the meniscus is dependent on the blood supply to the tissue, and the location of the tear. Because meniscus tears vary, so does recovery time and rehabilitative restrictions after surgery. Surgical options are as follows:

*Meniscectomy*: During a meniscectomy, only the torn portion of the meniscus is removed. Length of time for full recovery and return to function is approximately six to eight weeks.

*Meniscal Repair*: During a meniscal repair, the surgeon will repair the torn area of the meniscus with sutures. The ability to perform a meniscal repair is dependent on the type of tear and its location, but also on the age and athletic level of the patient. Recovery time is four to five months, and following surgery, range of motion will be limited to 45° to 90° of flexion within the first several weeks. The athlete will also be non-weight-bearing for four to six weeks.

Again, the postsurgical protocol is dependent on the type of procedure performed. A menisectomy will always have a shorter recovery since there is no time frame necessary to allow torn tissue to heal back into the bone. On the other hand, a meniscal repair, where the torn portion of the meniscus is physically sutured and anchored back into the bone, needs adequate time to heal back into the bone. There is no possible way to speed this up, and more limitations are placed on the athlete postoperatively in order to protect the graft.

### Prevention of Meniscus Injuries

Unfortunately, there is no true way to prevent a meniscus tear. As discussed previously, studies have shown that strengthening the quadriceps and hamstring muscle groups to promote lower body control can increase overall stability. This can certainly reduce the risk of meniscus tears, but once again, injury is an assumed risk in sport.

## PATELLAR DISLOCATIONS

Another common knee injury we see on the soccer field is the patellar dislocation or subluxation. The patella, or kneecap, is a sesamoid bone, which means it sits within a tendon; in this case, the distal quadriceps tendon. Its function is to work as a lever between the quadriceps and tibia or shin bone. The patella moves up and down within the trochlear groove of the femur during knee flexion and extension. The trochlear groove is made up of the distal femoral condyles, and makes up the medial and lateral borders surrounding the patella.

When the patella dislocates, it slips outside of the trochlear groove, most often to the lateral side. A higher incidence of this is seen in the female athlete, but can happen with the male athlete as well. The reason for this is again the larger Q-angle in females, which increases the lateral pull on the patella from the quadriceps.

### Signs and Symptoms of Patellar Dislocations

The most apparent symptom of a patellar subluxation is an obvious deformity, where the patella is malaligned. The athlete usually presents with a bent knee, and cannot extend or straighten the knee. Extreme pain and swelling can result. Based on this malalignment, the athlete will also not be able to walk or bear weight. With this type of presentation, it is very important that another player, coach, or parent, *does not rapidly extend the knee*! If an improper attempt to reduce the patella, that is, to put it back into place, is made, the patella can fracture. Please leave this to the medical professional to avoid turning this minor injury into a major one!

### Mechanism of Injury for Patellar Dislocations

Patellar subluxations can be caused by a direct impact to the knee, a twisting motion of the knee or ankle, or a sudden lateral cut. If an athlete has recurrent tightness in the tensor fasciae latae muscle (located on the outside of the upper thigh) or the IT band, or a quadriceps imbalance between the vastus lateralis and the vastus medialis, there is a higher risk of patellar dislocation. If there is an overactive vastus lateralis, or an underactive vastus medialis, there is an increased risk for a lateral slip. As mentioned above, patellar subluxations are more common in females, because their increased Q-angle contributes to some of these predisposing factors.

### Treatment of Patellar Dislocations

The patella often slides back into place on its own after subluxation, but if it does not, the first course of treatment is obviously to reduce the patella. Once back in place, it's a good idea to obtain an x-ray and make sure there is no fissuring or fracturing of the bone. Patellae that chronically sublux are at risk for secondary injuries to the posterior side, with small cracks or chips leading to a degenerative knee.

Following the initial trauma, the soccer player is now more susceptible to a second subluxation due to the instability of the trochlear joint and surrounding structures, namely the retinaculum, which is the band of tendons that holds the patella in place. Just like passing a button through the eyelet of a shirt is most difficult the first time, it will become easier and easier for the patella to pass through the retinaculum if it has been loosened up.

The physical therapist's first order of business is to decrease pain and swelling, then to return the knee to full range of motion. Once flexion and extension are pain-free to a full range of motion, the athlete can begin a progressive strengthening program.

This begins with muscle-setting exercises that focus on the VMO, or medial quad muscle, which directly affects the line of pull on the patella. Improving the strength and neuromuscular control of this muscle has shown benefits postinjury.

If there is no damage to the patellofemoral joint and the medial patellofemoral ligament is intact, the athlete can be back on the field within six to eight weeks. Of course, three to four weeks of strength training and conditioning are required prior to returning to the field.

### Prevention of Patellar Dislocations

To prevent patellar subluxations, the VMO needs to be as strong as possible. I think every running athlete, especially the adolescent soccer athlete, should utilize a good quadriceps and hamstring strengthening program.

Some athletes returning to play following a patellar subluxation will use a "J-brace" to further stabilize the knee. This knee sleeve has a bolster on the lateral side of the patella that can be tightened with Velcro. This will help to keep the patella from sliding laterally (see Figure 4.7).

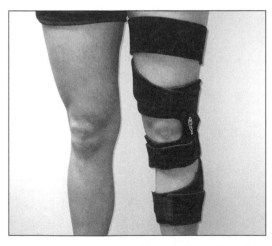

**Figure 4.7** J-strap knee brace: Stabilizes the patella within the trochlear groove. The strap is pulled in a lateral to medial direction.

# CHAPTER FIVE

# HIP AND THIGH INJURIES

As we move even further up the leg, we have now reached the hip and thigh complex. The hip joint is a ball-and-socket joint, also known as a spheroidal or multiaxial joint, in which the ball-shaped surface of one bone fits into the concave, cup-like depression of the other (see Figure 5.1). Unlike the knee joint, the hip joint is multidirectional, and can move across all three planes of motion: sagittal, frontal, and transverse. With running, kicking, and dribbling, the soccer athlete places a tremendous amount of demand on this joint. Combining the running movement with the explosive action of kicking, or with reaching out to stop a ball while maintaining a full sprint, requires a great amount of strength, flexibility, and control. The demands that soccer players place on their hip joints can lead to complex injuries in this area.

Like all joints in the body, the hip joint contains four types of tissue that hold together its structure: bones, ligaments, muscles, and tendons. The ligaments that hold together the pelvic bones extend into the proximal femur. Due to their location deep within

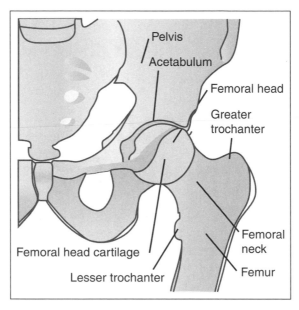

**Figure 5.1** Anatomy: Bones of the hip joint.

the musculature of the lumbo-pelvic-hip complex, or LPH, these structures are very rarely injured during athletic participation. The tendons, however, are the transmitters of action from the muscles to the bone. We will talk about some of the more important ones that often cause problems in the soccer athlete later on in this chapter.

Approximately 29 muscles make up the LPH complex, including the adductors, hamstrings, hip flexors, abdominals, erector spinae, tensor fascia latae, and gluteals. These muscles not only provide stability throughout the core, but also provide movement for the actions of running, jumping, and kicking. It is important to keep in mind the close relationship that exists between the joint, the bony junctions, and the many muscles in this area as injuries are treated, prevented, and rehabilitated. As with any joint, we can isolate specific musculature for rehabilitative purposes, but we must consider the multiplanar actions of the ball-and-socket joint and their impact on surrounding joints; namely, the spino-sacral junction and the lumbar spine.

## BIOMECHANICAL ANALYSIS OF THE LEG KICK

### Hip Extension, Abduction, and External Rotation

Let's look at the parallels between a pitcher's throwing motion and the soccer athlete's kicking motion (see Figure 5.2). In the early-cocking phase of pitching, the lead leg is planted firmly on the ground and the humerus (the long bone in the upper arm) is parallel to the ground and ready to achieve maximal external rotation at the shoulder. In what we'll consider the same phase in the soccer athlete, the lead leg is firmly planted on the ground, the kicking leg's femur is close to parallel with the ground and the hip is ready to achieve maximal hip extension, abduction, and external rotation; that is, the leg is extended backward and the hips are open to the side.

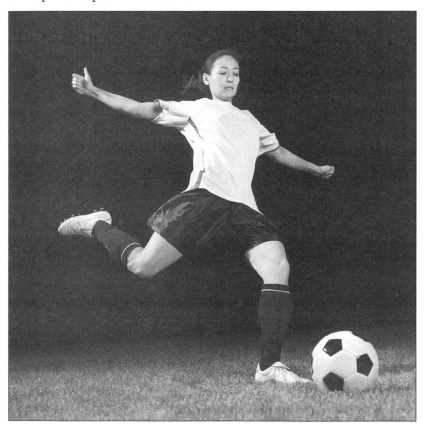

**Figure 5.2** Soccer athlete kicking ball.

We can consider this the loading phase, where the soccer athlete builds up as much potential energy as necessary to get the job done; that is, a max-effort leg drive to kick a ball all the way across the field, a soft touch into the box, or something in between. The muscle groups primarily responsible for this kind of leg action are the hamstrings and glutes, located on the posterior and lateral side of the hip. When these muscles fire, they shorten, creating potential energy in the antagonist muscle groups. Essentially, the firing of the hamstrings and glutes pre-loads the quadriceps and adductors for action.

### Hip Flexion, Adduction, and Internal Rotation

The combined movement of hip flexion and  adduction is important in the acceleration of the soccer athlete's lower leg in front of and across the body. Moving from an extended and abducted hip the leg accelerates to move from back to front, beginning with the core in a properly controlled movement that drives down and through the ball.

The most important hip flexor muscles are the rectus femoris and iliopsoas. Though the actions of these muscles are similar in their isolated function of hip flexion, in a dynamic leg swing or kick, the rectus femoris tends to take over, as it is a longer, larger, two-joint muscle.

Anatomically, the iliopsoas is a primary flexor of the hip. It originates at the lumbar spine, crosses the hip joint, and connects to the femur. The rectus femoris originates at the anterior superior iliac spine (the ASIS, which is the most prominent protuberance at the front of the hip) and inserts at the tibial tubercle by way of the patellar tendon. As mentioned, the rectus femoris is the longer of the two muscles, and it also acts in extending the knee. It is the rectus femoris that is most involved with the dynamic kicking motion, with the transferring of the force originating at the core, moving through the flexing hip, and exploding into a violent knee extension.

## MECHANISM OF INJURY FOR A MUSCLE STRAIN

When discussing injury  to these structures, we're often referring to a strain of the  musculature, which occurs when the muscle is stretched beyond its normal limit. This can be the result of doing too much too soon, inadequately warming-up or overworking the musculature, or it can simply be caused by a chance occurrence. As with most muscular injuries, the trauma can be either acute or chronic.

An acute muscle strain is the result of an immediate or sudden occurrence that causes pain. Most often this is from a rapid or violent kick when the athlete is in a fatigued or unprepared state. If it's early in the game or practice and the athlete decides to go at 100% before he or she is properly warmed-up, the muscles are not prepared for a rapid stretch-contraction. Conversely, when it's late in the game, and the athlete is dehydrated or fatigued, the muscle is also at risk for strain. So how do we find a happy medium?

Prior to athletic activity, we need to educate our athletes on proper ways to take care of and listen to their bodies. A proper warm-up progression during which the athlete breaks a sweat means he or she is getting adequate blood into the muscles. With improved blood flow, the muscles are actively being healed and increasing their extensibility, and thus their preparedness for activity.

Along with this activity, hydration is important to keep blood flowing smoothly through various tissues. Without enough fluid intake before, during, and after activity, blood becomes thicker and more viscous and has more difficulty traveling through the body. Aside from a clear drop in performance, this also puts the athlete at a greater risk for a muscle strain.

Chronic muscle strains are the result of the same motion, repeated over and over again. The same muscles are being worked in the same muscle pattern, relentlessly. Think about a kicker in American football. His job is extremely repetitive and does not allow for much diversity in training; a kicker only kicks, but think about how much more a typical soccer player kicks.

For soccer players, it's about proper management of their practice. Much like baseball pitchers keep a count on their pitches, soccer players must keep a count on their kicks. Their time should really be spent on good, quality reps, with a strong focus on technique. It doesn't make much sense for them to go out and kick until their legs are ready to fall off.

This is much the same way soccer athletes should be managed. The athlete should strive for quality repetitions over the course of each practice leading up to game day. This is especially true for the injured athlete returning back to the field.

## SIGNS AND SYMPTOMS OF MUSCLE STRAINS

Signs and symptoms of a muscle strain can range from a sharp, stabbing pain with activity to a basic ache during rest. There may be swelling, and most times there will be a visible, physical divot or spacing in the tissue. Depending on the severity or degree of the strain, you'll likely see a black and blue discoloration, combined with associated pain and loss of range of motion at either the knee or hip. When looking at more true tissue tears, such as a second- or third-degree tear, an orthopedic consult is necessary.

## DEGREES OF MUSCLE TEARS

**First Degree:** Overstretch of muscle fibers

**Second Degree:** Tearing of a few fibers

**Third Degree:** Full tear of the musculature.

It's often difficult to distinguish among the different strains without some sort of advanced imaging that can directly see and define how much tearing actually occurred. But ultimately, the same treatment will be utilized regardless of degree to relieve the athlete of discomfort, reduce inflammation, and protect from further damage. With any strain, it's not always beneficial to immediately see a physician as long as the athlete is being properly treated. Persistent symptoms and lack of improvement over the course of four to seven days may warrant further medical intervention.

## ADDUCTOR STRAIN

There are four adductor muscles that extend from the pubic bone to the femur; the adductor magnus, minimus, brevis, and longus (see Figure 5.3). They function to bring the leg across the body, as seen in the actions of passing, shooting, and lateral motion.

An adductor strain can occur very often in the soccer athlete, and is unique in that the area of injury has a high rate of differential diagnoses. Basically, what this means is that there are a lot of different things that can be going on in that region, so it's

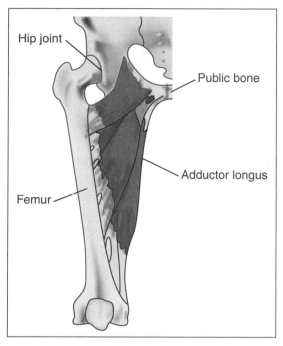

**Figure 5.3** Anatomy: Adductor muscle group.

important to rule out other injuries, such as a sports hernia or athletic pubalgia, labral tear, hip flexor strain, or pubitis (which is inflammation between the pubic bones), prior to diagnosing an adductor strain.

Actions that may cause pain to an athlete with an adductor strain are side-to-side motion, especially when shifting direction and trying to pass the ball. Keep in mind that it's not just the motion of adduction we need to limit, but also abduction of the hip that will cause a stretch to this musculature. As described above, this is where you bring your leg all the way out to the side, and all the way in while winding up to kick the ball as hard as possible.

## HAMSTRING STRAIN

Depending on the location of the damaged structures, hamstring strains are usually felt in the middle of the posterior thigh. Because the length of the hamstring muscle group covers the entire back of the thigh, you can strain this muscle in any area.

The hamstring originates at the ischium, which is the portion of the pelvic bone that we sit on, and attaches all the way down at the tibia and fibula (see Figure 5.4). There are two medial hamstring muscles, known as the semitendinosus and semimembranosus. The biceps femoris is located on the lateral side, and is made up of two heads leading to a singular insertion. These large muscle bellies make up the posterior thigh musculature, with the tendons running distally, making up the borders of the space behind the knee with their corresponding tendon location. An overstretch can strain one of these three muscles acutely, with the biceps femoris being the most often strained.

The hamstring acts at both the hip and knee joints and is primarily responsible for hip extension and knee flexion. Because the hamstring is so utilized during soccer activities like running and kicking, the continual fatigue factor comes into play with regard to injury. Hamstring strains are very common among soccer athletes and cause a tremendous amount of games lost to injury at all levels.

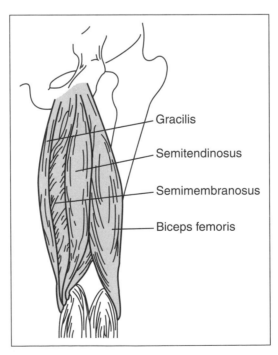

**Figure 5.4** Anatomy: Hamstring muscle group.

## QUADRICEPS STRAIN

The quadriceps muscle grouping on the anterior portion of the thigh includes four powerful muscles that act to flex the hip and extend the knee: the vastus medialis, vastus lateralis, vastus intermedius, and rectus femoris (see Figure 5.5). Like the hamstring, the quadriceps also crosses two joints, acting as the primary knee extender as well as supporting hip flexion. Of course, actions are different, but these muscles are all strained in the same manner when the muscles are stretched beyond their normal limits.

## TREATMENT OF MUSCLE STRAINS

Most soccer players try to come back from muscle strains way too quickly, and do not understand the importance of rest. As discussed previously, any type of strained muscle should be treated with the RICE protocol. Instinctively, most people will try to stretch or roll out their muscle on a foam roller to alleviate their pain. This is *not*

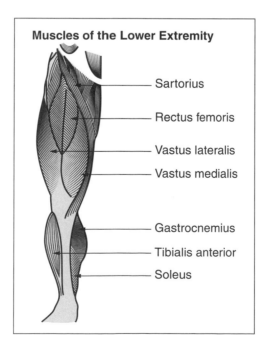

**Muscles of the Lower Extremity**

Sartorius

Rectus femoris

Vastus lateralis

Vastus medialis

Gastrocnemius

Tibialis anterior

Soleus

**Figure 5.5** Anatomy: Quadriceps muscle group.

recommended for the acute strain! Although these can be beneficial treatment options, they should not be performed until the muscle has had a chance to recover and heal. Before progressing into any type of functional rehab and certainly before returning to running or playing, the muscle must heal down.

### So When Can I Stretch a Strained Muscle?

When I see an athlete with a muscle strain, I try to decrease pain and swelling through simple things such as anti-inflammatory medication (NSAID) modalities, and icing. I make sure the athlete can walk without pain before progressing the rehab. Usually, the initial goals are to decrease inflammation and pain, restore normal function of the hip, and restore knee range of motion.

Sometimes, the athlete will have to be non-weight-bearing with a compression bandage at the beginning of his or her treatment. With this situation, it is important to understand that the muscle must heal prior to any progression to flexibility.

Once the athlete can walk, sit, and stand without pain, he or she can begin to progress into some low-level flexibility protocols (see Figure 5.6). Included with this plan should be a strength

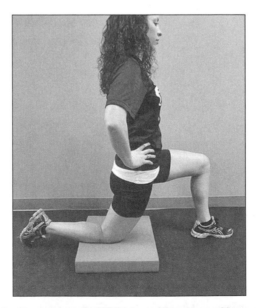

**Figure 5.6** Hip flexor stretch: While kneeling on an Airex pad, press the right hip forward, slightly arching the low back.

progression beginning with muscle-setting exercises and advancing to more functional components.

As with all rehab, it is not about just the injury, but the entire limb, taking into account the joints above and below the injury. As the patient starts to regain strength, he or she can then progress into closed kinetic chain activities. Follow those with sport-specific activities, including plyometrics, ultimately with a full return to play.

## RUNNING PROTOCOL FOLLOWING A MUSCLE STRAIN

Once a full range of motion is achieved with good baseline strength, the athlete can begin a running program that includes running straight ahead, backpedalling, running diagonally, and shuffling. When the athlete can run with no pain, he or she can advance into more soccer-specific drills, such as dribbling and passing, with a full return back to sport. The idea with any return-to-play protocol is to break down each movement to the micro-level, and rebuild the athlete from the ground up, restoring foundational movements first, and then progressing to larger, macro-level activities.

With a muscle strain, there is really no specific return-to-sport protocol outside of the general guidelines of hitting key benchmarks prior to advancing to the next. Time frames are all dependent on how well the individual athlete is progressing through the rehab. No two injuries are the same and each should be treated individually.

Throughout rehab, it's important to keep in mind the biomechanics of the muscle. Know that certain activities will stress, stretch, or strain certain areas of the body in very specific ways. Before even engaging in certain activities, think about the movement and assess whether or not the activity will aggravate the injury. Each athlete must listen to his or her body and not do anything that will cause discomfort. A little TLC in the recovery phase will go a long way later on down the road.

## PREVENTION OF HIP AND THIGH MUSCLE STRAINS

To prevent muscle strains in the hip and thigh, we need to take into account the dynamic component of what a soccer player does, along with how we use our thigh musculature throughout our normal daily activities. Our hips are being flexed all day long, not just while we're playing soccer. Common symptoms of hip and thigh muscle strains will consist of anterior hip pain, exacerbated when going up and down stairs or walking. It is important that we strengthen the muscles in our hips and thighs, and include hip flexor, core, pelvic stabilization, and flexibility exercises in our training program. Remember, if the hip flexor doesn't work, playing in a soccer game is going to be a very difficult task.

Sometimes athletic trainers will attempt what's known as a *hip spica* (see Figure 5.7). This is essentially a prophylactic bracing, where an ace wrap is wrapped around the thigh and waist in a manner that assists the muscle action and alleviates pain. This can be done to support a hamstring or hip flexor or adductor strain. Depending on the injury location, positional shortening of the musculature followed by the wrapping technique will assist the musculature during physical activity. This

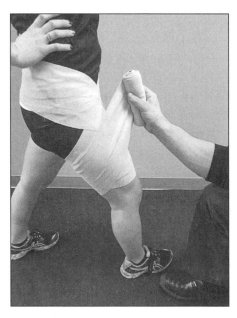

**Figure 5.7** Hip spica: This athletic prophylactic uses an Ace wrap to mimic the action of the hip flexor muscle group. The injured hip is placed in standing flexion and slight internal rotation to shorten the muscle while applying the wrap.

doesn't always work for the athlete, and it is dependent on the severity of injury, stage of return to play, and the intensity of their action as an athlete.

As with all muscular injuries, prevention of muscle strains in the hip and thigh is quite simple. The muscle needs to be strong enough to handle the demands of the sport. Good training and conditioning, along with a good warm-up, are pivotal components of any athlete's fitness routine. Of course, early intervention with an injury can truly reduce the time away from the field. Remember that a first-degree strain can quickly turn into a second- or third-degree strain without appropriate care and attention.

**THE WARM-UP**

As we've talked about throughout this book, the importance of a good warm-up cannot be understated. A warm-up does not consist of a two-minute jog around the field. The purpose of the warm-up is to generate good blood flow within key musculature that we're going to need for our practice or game, and is definitively sport- and position-specific.

A good rule of thumb is that the athlete should be sweating prior to engaging in more dynamic athletic activity. Depending on the athlete's sport and position, different musculature is used more often than others.

If you look at the end-lines of any Major League Soccer game, you will see a group of players continually moving through a circuit of light jogging and agility drills designed to keep their legs warm and ready for action. These athletes know their bodies well enough to understand that they cannot just jump into the game directly from the bench. Staying loose and flexible will keep them ready to go at a moment's notice and, most importantly, will keep them safe from injury.

**QUAD CONTUSION**

A quad contusion, or bruise, is the result of a direct impact to the muscle. The soccer athlete most often suffers a quad contusion when going up for 50/50 headers, where one athlete will knee the other soccer player directly into the quad muscle group. The direct blow will likely cause broken blood vessels and subcutaneous bleeding. Once this happens, blood will pool in the area. Although most often mild, quad contusions can be quite painful, and if not treated properly, can actually result in a calcification of the muscle known as myositis ossificans.

Myositis ossificans can be explained by looking at its name: the muscle (myo) ossifies, or forms bone, resulting in a lack of mobility and flexibility within the quad muscle group. In order to properly treat this, we have to instill a protocol of RICE and flexibility! The athletic trainer or physical therapist may want to use electrical stimulation to help with pain control as well, but the most important components at play here are icing to decrease the blood pooling in the area and stretching to maintain the flexibility of the muscle.

There are two things we *never* want to do when treating myositis ossificans. First, we don't want a second impact to be suffered during play, so proper padding is required. Second, we don't want to apply moist heat as we often want to do with muscular injuries. With any acute trauma, the body will initiate its own inflammatory response, bringing fluid to the area. Moist heat will only increase the fluid volume and hasten cellular death, while icing and stretching will combat those symptoms.

As stated above, these cases are usually mild, but can be classified more severely based on the symptoms of pain, swelling, stiffness, and loss of function (see Figure 5.8).

## ATHLETIC PUBALGIA

Although not one of the most common injuries, soccer athletes do encounter athletic pubalgia, also known as a sports hernia, which is a pain syndrome of the anterior abdomen. In males, pain will spread into the testicles and distally around the pubic bone, causing a deep ache with increased motion. Physicians' opinions differ on what causes athletic pubalgia: some have identified it as a tissue tear, most commonly of the inguinal ligament; others have identified it as an issue of adductor dysfunction; and still others have identified it as an impingement of the femoral nerve. As someone that practices soccer medicine, I think it is important

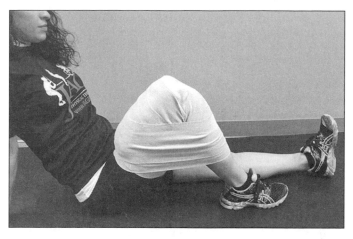

**Figure 5.8** Quad contusion ice and stretch: Place an ice pack directly over the contusion and wrap an ACE wrap around the thigh and shin to keep the knee in supported flexion.

to rule out hip issues prior to checking for a sports hernia. Many hip pathologies, such as labral tears, hip flexor or adductor tears, or a femoroacetabular impingement can elicit symptoms similar to those of athletic pubalgia. Athletes suffering from pain in the pelvis should be seen by an orthopedic surgeon to identify the true cause of their pain.

## INTERNAL SNAPPING HIP SYNDROME

Snapping hip syndrome is characterized by an audible snap or click within or around the hip joint, along with a popping sensation felt internally. It is caused when the iliopsoas muscle becomes thick and swollen and catches on the greater trochanter, or femoral head, as the hip is flexed. Soccer players who suffer from internal snapping hip syndrome will experience this popping and the accompanying discomfort every time they run down field.

Deep-tissue massage to increase the extensibility of the iliopsoas muscle belly is a good way to treat internal snapping hip syndrome, but it can be uncomfortable for the athlete due to the muscle's location deep within the abdomen. It should be done by a physical therapist or athletic trainer. Moist heat at the front of the hip can also be beneficial, as can stretching exercises for the hip flexor.

## LABRUM TEARS

The hip joint is another ball-and-socket joint with articulations between the femur and pelvis, with the femoral head being the ball and the pelvis the socket. This allows for a larger range of motion at our hips. The labrum is a layer of cartilage at the articular surface of the pelvis that provides added stability to the femoral head as it sits in this groove. The labrum also provides a smooth surface for the gliding of the bones against one another.

Much of the actual stability at the hip joint is provided by the massive amount of musculature in the area. Many muscles, including the glutes, hamstrings, quadriceps, psoas, tensor fascia latae, and many other small rotators originate at the pelvis and attach at the femur; remember, there are 29 individual muscles that make up the lumbo-pelvic-hip complex! So, while there is a tremendous amount of range of motion at the hip, there is also a lot holding it in place.

A final important detail to consider in this joint is the shape and orientation of the femoral neck and head. Although this ball-and-socket joint is similar to the shoulder in many ways, a major difference is the femoral neck as it angles into the pelvis. The orientation can vary in all three planes of motion: frontal, sagittal, and transverse. Subsequently, the femoral head can have various dynamics as it articulates with the pelvis. Depending on the mechanics of the insertion of the femoral head, as well as its shape (no one's is perfectly round like an actual ball!), some people have a higher risk for injury to the labrum or surrounding structures.

### Mechanism of Injury for Labrum Tears

As with most other injuries discussed thus far, there is a difference in the acute versus chronic mechanism of labral tears.

Acute labral tears most often occur with a dislocated or subluxated hip; a subluxation is a dislocation with a rapid, spontaneous reduction. That is, the hip pops out and then goes back in. Although rare due to the large amount of musculature holding the hip joint in place, this injury can occur as a result of a violent force with high velocity, and can result in trauma not only to the labrum, but to the surrounding structures as well. Please note that a hip dislocation is a medical emergency, and should be treated as such, because the blood supply to the lower limb can be compromised. The possibility of the occluding or obstruction of an artery supplying the leg is very real, and must be treated with care. Never should anyone attempt to relocate or reduce a dislocated hip on the field. This should be done under the care of a physician at a trauma center, where proper equipment is available.

As a result of the trauma of the femur sliding out of its natural articulation with the hip socket, there may be a tear in the labrum. A true diagnosis of a labrum tear is confirmed with an MRI-arthrogram, where dye is injected into the hip for an accurate depiction of the joint structures, which are difficult to discern on a regular MRI. A radiologist will confirm the diagnosis from the images taken and determine the degree of tear, ranging in severity from a mild grade 1 to a most-problematic grade 4.

Chronic labral tears are caused by repeated insult to the labrum. This can be the result of an anatomical deformity or abnormality in the way the femoral head is shaped or articulates with the hip socket, which causes unusual wearing and tearing of the joint cartilage. For soccer athletes, the twisting, rotating, flexing, and extending of the hip involved on a daily basis are unavoidable. It may not stop us from playing, but it can cause a degeneration of the labrum.

**Signs snd Symptoms of Labral Tears**

Most often, an athlete with a labrum tear will present to an athletic trainer complaining of anterior hip pain. Because there are a number of tissues in the area that could be the source of the pain, it is always important to rule out any intra-articular hip pathology prior to confirming any other diagnoses. In this instance, the labrum is the intra-articular hip pathology we are most often looking for. Athletes will present with painful ranges of motion, possibly describing a click or a catch in the groin that comes and goes. Groin strains can often be misdiagnosed as a labrum tear, and a labrum tear can often be misdiagnosed as a groin strain. An MRI-arthrogram is necessary for a proper diagnosis.

### Treatment of Labral Tears

Initially, athletic trainers and physical therapists will often treat the labrum conservatively, first utilizing the RICE protocol to limit inflammation. Due to the multiple muscular attachments in the area and the possibility of tight musculature leading to pain, manual therapy techniques can often be helpful in treating less severe causes. Unfortunately with a labrum, there are only so many treatment techniques and options available in a rehabilitation setting. Ultimately, it comes down to the athlete's level of discomfort and ability to compete at a high level. The labrum cannot heal itself, but pain can be managed in a variety of ways, including NSAIDs and steroid injections.

As pain is always the best subjective guideline, if pain persists, and treatment is no longer yielding improvements, it is time for the athlete to follow up with a physician and see what their options are moving forward.

### Surgical Intervention

If conservative treatment options have been exhausted, surgical intervention may be necessary. Depending on the cause and extent of the labral tear, the surgeon can either excise, or remove, the torn piece of labrum or repair the torn tissue by sewing it back together. Depending on the anatomy and mechanism of injury, there may be different tweaks to the procedure to reduce the risk of recurrence. Such things might involve shaving down an abnormal extension off the femur that is destroying the cartilage.

However the surgeon decides to repair the joint, a specific treatment plan will be detailed to protect the acutely repaired hip. Following surgery, it can be upwards of six months before the athlete is ready to return to the field, but there is a good success rate with labral repair surgery.

**Prevention of Labral Tears**

Prevention of labral tears often comes from the inclusion of good strength, flexibility, and balance components in a training regimen. Making sure the athlete has equal strength and control on both sides of their body is key. Doing the right stretches to keep the hips flexible and mobile is also beneficial. As with any injury, early intervention is often helpful in limiting or deterring insult to tissue.

# CHAPTER SIX

# SPINAL INJURIES

The cervical spine consists of seven vertebral segments, beginning at the base of the skull and interlocking on their way down the axial skeleton toward the trunk. These irregular-shaped bones encapsulate the spinal cord as it extends from the brain stem all the way down to the tips of the fingers and toes. Aside from protecting the spinal cord, the cervical spine also allows freedom of motion in all four planes. The ligaments and musculature that surround the cervical spine support this free range of motion.

When soccer players suffer injuries to the cervical spine, they are most often injuries to the musculoskeletal system. Whether a strain, sprain, or spasm, the injury often occurs as the result of a sudden, unexpected twist or turn, or what is commonly referred to as "whiplash." Proper neck strength is important, not only to control and support the head, but to protect it from injury.

Although soccer players are mainly running athletes, they do use their upper extremities during the course of play. Though against the rules, pulling at or grabbing another player, pushing off another player, or falling to the ground may cause injury. However, in the majority of cases when a soccer player injures his or her cervical spine, it is as a result of a headed ball.

## BIOMECHANICS OF THE HEADER

The proper form to prevent injury to the head and neck is to *brace for impact* (see figure 6.1). A retraction of the scapula and flexing of the trapezium allows a soccer player to brace for impact while transferring maximal force through the upper back and spine. This is an important skill to practice, especially for the young soccer athlete who may not have prominent or well-developed neck musculature. The best way to begin is through simple drills allowing the athlete to work on form outside of a game or practice situation.

### Trapezius Muscle

The trapezius is a rather large muscle that originates at the protuberance at the back of the skull, extends outwardly to the back of the shoulders, and inserts down at the thoracic and even lumbar spine. It is mostly superficial and different segments of the muscle contribute to head extension and shoulder shrugging. Mainly, the purpose of the trapezius as a whole is to prevent the head from falling forward due to gravity. In soccer, it serves to brace the head and neck for impact. When the trapezius is in a fully flexed position, the head is pulled back and the shoulders are shrugged up toward the ears.

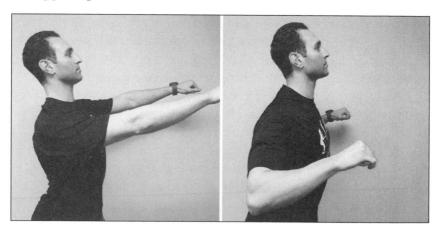

**Figure 6.1** Proper biomechanics of the header: Brace for impact by retracting the scapulae, shrugging the shoulders and tightening the muscles of the neck. Keep the mouth closed and try to make contact with the ball with the center of the forehead, at the natural hairline. Always move your head to the ball, don't wait for it to hit you.

### The Sternocleidomastoid Muscle (SCM)

Don't be intimidated by the lengthy name of this muscle, because its function is quite simple and well-defined by its name. This long muscle originates at the mastoid process (the protuberance directly behind your ear), extends down the side of the neck to the proximal clavicle, or collar bone (cleido-) and inserts at the superior sternum, or breastbone (sterno-). The SCM is involved with the flexion, extension, and rotation of the skull on the axis of the vertebra. To demonstrate the function of this muscle, place one finger behind the ear and another at the superior sternum, and use the head to bring the two fingers together. The head will twist downward and laterally. That is the action of the SCM.

There is one SCM on each side of the neck. Repeat this exercise on the other side, then try to do both at the same time. What happens? The head comes down toward the chest. When these two muscles act together, they work to flex the head down in such a manner, much like the action needed for a good strong header on the soccer field.

### COMMON MUSCULAR INJURIES OF THE CERVICAL SPINE

The trapezius and the SCM are the two most commonly strained muscles of the cervical spine. As is true with any strained muscle, we worry about the acuteness and severity of the strain (first, second, or third degree). Because of the strength and size of the musculature, it is uncommon to see anything beyond a first- or second-degree strain in sport. Certainly, more traumatic injuries, such as car accidents, are capable of causing a more severe strain, but they are generally not seen in athletics.

The trapezius is the more often injured of the two muscles. Athletes will often describe a sharp, burning pain, midway between the neck and shoulder. This is usually the result of a soccer athlete falling to the ground after going shoulder-to-shoulder with another player. A possible rolling of the neck, or sharp sudden twist without contact, can also result in injury.

While bruising does occasionally accompany a trapezius strain, the most common symptoms are an inflamed muscle that is painful to the touch and stiffness in the movements of the neck.

## Treatment of Common Muscular Injuries of the Cervical Spine

The first goal in treating a strained neck muscle is to decrease pain and dysfunction as quickly as possible, followed by a restoration of range of motion (see Figure 6.2). In the acute injury, ice is important to reduce pain and limit the inflammatory response, and it is often necessary to be taken out of the game for rest. Depending on the presentation of the acute injury, it is crucial for the on-site medical personnel to rule out any possible trauma resulting in damage to the cervical spine or spinal cord. On-field assessment of the traumatically injured athlete is beyond the scope of this book, but keep in mind that the on-site athletic trainer or EMT is responsible for directing care in the emergently injured athlete.

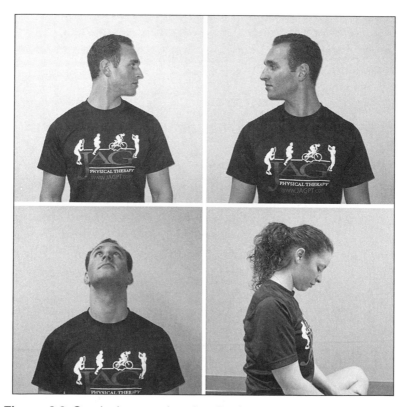

**Figure 6.2** Cervical range of motion: Basic range of motion test to rule out any painful sensations or lack of mobility in the cervical spine. Includes rotation and bending to both sides, flexion and extension.

Once the athlete is assessed for any further type of injury, and truly diagnosed with a strain, the athlete will start with a physical therapist or athletic trainer for therapeutic exercise to restore strength and mobility while allowing the body to heal with physical rest. Modalities such as ice, anti-inflammatory medication, and electric stimulation are good for this phase of rehabilitation. Beginning range of motion exercises will include flexion, extension, side-bending, and rotation.

After full range of motion is restored in the neck, the athlete can begin exercises to restore good strength to the muscle. This is done with simple isometrics so as not to tax the cervical spine. Football or wrestling athletes are often seen doing head and neck exercises with a weight strapped around their head, or with aggressive towel resistance, but this is not generally recommend because the added load increases the risk for rupturing a spinal disc.

Aside from good isometric strengthening, upper body exercises such as the upright row or shrugs can help increase the strength of the trapezius muscle. Certain Olympic lifts, such as the power clean, can also be beneficial, as they incorporate these motions as part of the bigger movement.

### Prevention of Common Muscular Injuries of the Cervical Spine

Of course, it is impossible to prevent all collisions in a contact sport like soccer. But the easiest way to prevent a muscular strain in the cervical spine is through good education at an early age that will provide an understanding of how to properly head the ball. Good head and neck control, along with the development of the necessary strength of all the neck musculature, will considerably reduce the risk of injury.

### DISC HERNIATION OF THE CERVICAL SPINE

More aggressive cervical injuries that can affect the soccer player include the herniation, or bulging, of the intervertebral disc (see Figure 6.3). Discs are often likened to jelly donuts; each one is made up of an outer band called the annulus fibrosus that surrounds a gel-like substance called the nucleus pulposus.

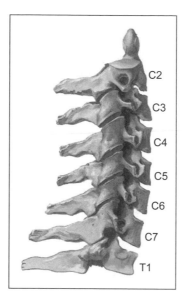

**Figure 6.3** Anatomy: Cervical vertebrae.

When a disc is herniated, the outer band is cracked or broken and the gel inside the disc leaks through into the spinal canal and can place pressure on the spinal cord.

This injury will strongly mimic that of a cervical strain, with similar signs and symptoms of pain, burning, and inflammatory response. The most common distinguishing factor is pain, numbness, and tingling extending down into the shoulder and arm. This is known as a cervical radiculopathy, where an impingement, entrapment, or pinch of the nerve is caused when a portion of the disc is in physical contact with the nerve root as it extends from the vertebrae. This can be identified through a physical exam that tests the strength and sensation in the upper extremities.

In soccer, a cervical disk herniation is most often caused by trauma from a collision with another athlete or with the ground or turf. The onset of symptoms is rapid. Muscular weakness is a common symptom associated with cervical disk herniations at the C5-C6 and C6-C7 levels, at the middle of the neck, where the vertebrae are more exposed and vulnerable. Based on their more protected position at the base of the skull, it is very rare to herniate a disk between C1 and C4 in an athletic setting (see Figure 6.4).

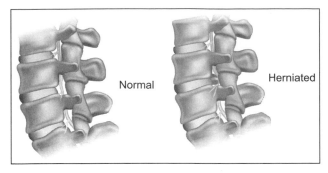

Normal

Herniated

**Figure 6.4** Anatomy: Disc herniation of the cervical vertebrae.

### Four Stages of Disc Herniation

**Disc Degeneration:** Chemical changes, often associated with age, cause the discs to weaken but not protrude.

**Prolapse:** The shape or position of the disc changes and creates a slight impingement into the spinal canal. Also called a protrusion or a bulging disc.

**Extrusion:** The gel-like nucleus pulposus breaks through the wall of the disc but remains within the disc.

**Sequestration:** The nucleus pulposus breaks through the wall of the disc and spills into the spinal canal.

### Treatment of Disc Herniations of the Cervical Spine

These types of injuries can be treated by your physical therapist or athletic trainer with rest, modalities, and forms of traction to relieve pressure and inflammation. An anti-inflammatory medication, such as ibuprofen, can also be used. All soccer players suspected to have these types of injuries must see a physician immediately so the severity of the herniation can be evaluated.

Usually the physician and the physical therapist will wait for symptoms to resolve before progressing the athlete back to range-of-motion and functional strengthening activities. If the athlete is able to achieve a sport-specific routine, then he or she may be cleared for the collision sport of soccer. If symptoms do not resolve in an appropriate time, the physician might consider a more invasive treatment, such as an epidural steroid injection, or, in extreme cases, a surgical intervention.

The only way to prevent cervical disk herniations is to make sure the body is strong enough to handle the demands of the sport. Proper biomechanics and direction on how to head a ball should also be taken into consideration. General upper extremity strengthening is important for a soccer player to remain safe and reduce the risk of injury (see Figures 6.5 and 6.6).

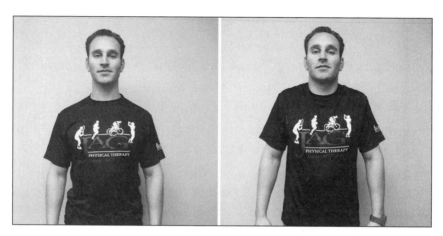

**Figure 6.5** Shoulder shrugs: Standing with good posture, engage the trapezius muscles to elevate the shoulders up toward the ears.

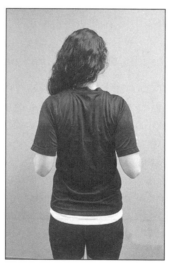

**Figure 6.6** Scapular retraction: Scapular strengthening exercise that places the shoulder blades in proper upright position and prevents forward-tilting (kyphotic) posture. Squeeze the shoulder blades together toward the spine.

## "BURNERS" AND "STINGERS" IN THE BRACHIAL PLEXUS

The brachial plexus is a very important component of the cervical spine, as it relates to the function of the shoulder, arm, and hand. The brachial plexus is a network of nerve fibers that extends off the spinal cord from vertebral segments C5-T1, and separates into nerve roots, trunks, divisions, and cords as they extend the neurological supply to the upper extremities.

Injuries to the brachial plexus are most often referred to as "burners" or "stingers." These are the result of a stretch of the brachial plexus as it extends out of the neck into the shoulder, which interferes with the nerve supply to the upper arm. A forceful rotation of the head away from the shoulder, often with the arm extended, can cause transient neurological symptoms. Burners and stingers are most often temporary and will resolve with proper rest. The specific amount of rest needed is dependent on the severity of injury, and the athlete's history with it. Athletes with a history of chronic injuries to the brachial plexus are at risk for long-term deficits in strength and sensation.

Testing of the brachial plexus is fairly simple, with a choreographed examination that tests the sensory and motor nerves of the upper extremity. These tests reveal any transient deficits in strength or sensation that are indicators of neurologic dysfunction. A reproduction of symptoms can often be elicited with a brachial plexus stretch test (see Figure 6.7), and is a strong indicator of this injury.

On the following page is a chart of the different nerve roots and their innervations, which make up the brachial plexus. Damage to each specific nerve root can cause symptoms in specific areas supplied by each spinal nerve, known as dermatomes. There are eight cervical nerves that originate at the cervical vertebrae. The first thoracic vertebrae, T1, is the transitional vertebrae between the cervical spine and the thoracic spine and is included.

A myotome is a specific area of musculature innervated by the various nerve roots as they branch off the spinal cord. Each myotome is responsible for specific muscular actions, as defined in the chart on page 109.

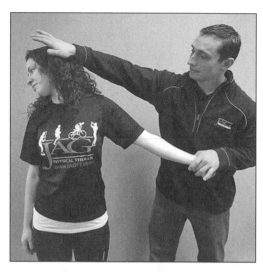

**Figure 6.7** Brachial plexus stretch test: While tilting the head away from the shoulder, simultaneously extend and externally rotate the arm, placing the brachial plexus into a stretch. This exercise often reproduces symptoms consistent with a brachial plexus injury.

| DERMATOME | SENSATION |
|---|---|
| C1 & C2 | Top of skull |
| C3 | Temporal bones |
| C4 | Sides of neck |
| C5 | Acromion process (tip of shoulder) |
| C6 | Outer arm down to thumb |
| C7 | Mid-forearm to middle finger |
| C8 | Medial forearm to fifth finger |
| T1 | Medial humerus |

These same symptoms apply to a cervical disc herniation. A brachial plexus injury is a stretch of the nerve root that only has transient effects that will dissipate fairly rapidly, while a herniation is more of a mechanical malfunction that takes more time to resolve; the phrase, "you can't put the jelly back in the donut" is common. Once you herniate a disc, it cannot fully heal. But it can be excised by a surgeon.

It should be noted that just because you have this diagnosis does not mean you will have all of the symptoms described.

| MYOTOME | MOTOR ACTION |
|---------|--------------|
| C1 & C2 | Neck flexion |
| C3 | Lateral neck flexion |
| C4 | Shoulder shrugging |
| C5 | Shoulder abduction |
| C6 | Elbow extension and wrist flexion |
| C7 | Elbow flexion and wrist extension |
| C8 | Thumb abduction and ulnar deviation |
| T1 | Finger abduction and adduction |

These are only indicators of the injury, and proper evaluation by a physician, who will likely prescribe an MRI, will reveal the exact cause of your discomfort.

Burners and stingers typically resolve on their own, within 20 minutes. If symptoms persist, seek the help of a medical professional. Persistent injuries to the brachial plexus are most commonly treated conservatively, with strengthening and flexibility protocols for the neck and trapezius.

## LUMBAR SPINE INJURIES

Regardless of whether or not they are soccer players, or even athletes of any kind, thousands of Americans suffer from lower back injuries. In a normal, healthy individual, the lumbar spine curves in an anterior to posterior direction; if you look at the lumbar spine from the side, the curve is slightly concave (see Figure 6.8). Because the human body likes to be in balance, if there is a sway too far in one direction, there is always a corrective sway in the opposing direction. This gives us balance in our upright posture, and allows us improved functionality throughout our daily activities.

However, excess curvature in the spine can lead to kyphotic or lordotic curvature. Lordosis, or swayback, is a condition in which the spine in the lower back is excessively curved, putting extra pressure on the spine and causing pain. Kyphosis is an exaggerated rounding of the upper back, sometimes referred to as a hunchback.

Certain body types are more prone to an exacerbation of the curvature of the spine, or conversely, a lack there-of, causing problems above and below that area of the spine.

## Causes of Lumbar Spine Injuries

### *Lumbar Strains*

Soccer athletes are running athletes who have to run and kick a ball simultaneously, which puts stress on the lower extremities. They also commonly use one side of their body much more often than the other, and that repetitive overuse on a single side

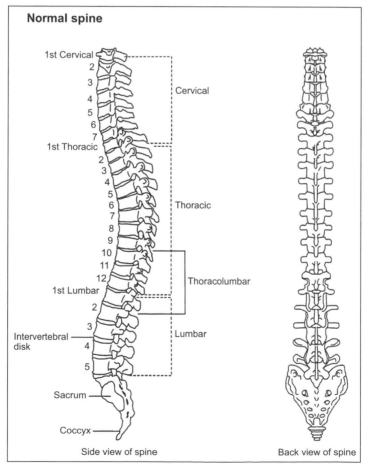

**Figure 6.8** Anatomy: Lateral view of the spine.

*Source*: Image courtesy of the National Institute of Arthritis and Musculoskeletal and Skin Diseases.

of the body can often lead to weakness on the opposite side. For a variety of reasons, soccer players often suffer lumbar strains to the variety of tiny muscles that run along both sides of the spine. Lumbar strains often result in lower back spasms.

The pain caused by a lumbar comes on quickly and can be accompanied with loss of motion, loss of strength, and the inability to flex, extend, and rotate the trunk.

Lower back spasms are generally the result of the spinal vertebrae being out of position (see Figure 6.9). While back pain can sometimes be caused by problems in the back, it is more often the result of a dysfunction in the structures that attach directly to the lumbar spine and pelvis. It is important to determine the actual cause of the back pain, and treat it directly.

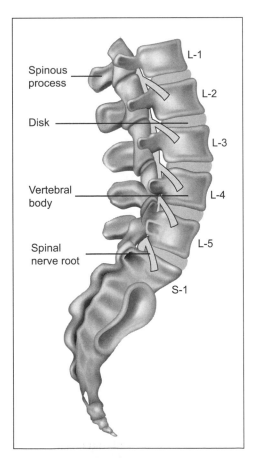

**Figure 6.9** Anatomy: Lumbar vertebrae.

### Hamstring Group

The hamstring muscles attach on the inferior portion of the pelvis, and due to their location on the posterior, tend to have pull in that direction. An athlete with "tight hamstrings" will have difficulties with the entire posterior chain. This athlete will often present with a "flat back," which occurs when the hamstrings are so tight they pull the pelvis backwards, flattening out the normal curve in the lower back. This leads to a weakening of the quadriceps and back muscles, and may cause back pain.

### Quadriceps/Hip Flexor Group

The quadriceps and hip flexors attach directly to the anterior pelvis and lumbar spine. Tightness in this muscle grouping will lead to an anterior pull on the pelvis, and an increased lordotic curve, which can also cause back pain.

### Treatment of Lumbar Strains

After you have determined that you are dealing with a lumbar strain, the first step of treatment is the RICE protocol, as seen on page 4. I suggest a consult with a physician to rule out any type of herniation, spondylolysis, or stress fracture of the vertebrae.

It is also important to test for any radiculopathy that may be present, so more serious injury can be ruled out. If there is no radiculopathy, we can assume the pain is local and most likely the result of a strain or sprain. This can easily be rehabilitated by a physical therapist or athletic trainer, with the utilization of modalities such as electrical stimulation and moist heat, and by increasing flexibility of the hamstrings, quadriceps, glutes, and paraspinal muscles, which run parallel to and support the spine. In addition to a good flexibility program, a good core-strengthening program can also help treat and prevent lower back pain (see Figures 6.10–6.12).

These same exercises can be used in a good prevention program that can reduce the risk of injury. Other ways to prevent lower back spasms are to incorporate a good warm-up prior to activity and cool-down after activity that include a flexibility routine that targets problem areas. If the hamstrings or quads are tight, stretch them.

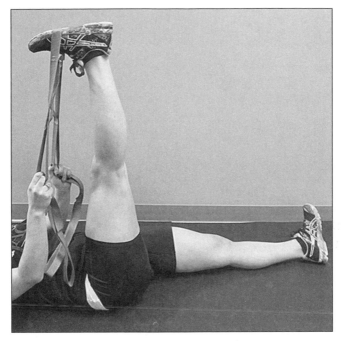

**Figure 6.10** Supine hamstring stretch: While lying on your back, place a strap or belt around the foot and elevate it toward the ceiling with your arms. Pull the strap back toward your face, keeping the leg straight.

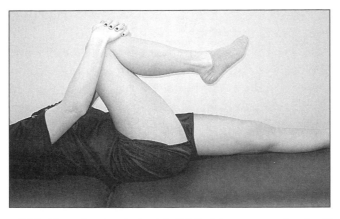

**Figure 6.11** Knee-to-chest stretch: While lying on your back with your legs out in front of you, pull your knees to your chest, one at a time, stretching your lower back. Hold for 30 seconds. Repeat three times on each side.

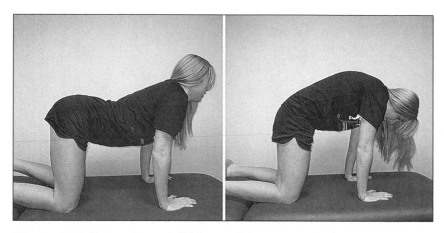

**Figure 6.12** Cat and camel: While on all fours, round your back up toward the ceiling until you feel a stretch in the upper, middle, and lower back. Hold for 10 seconds. Return to a flat back, then press your stomach toward the floor and tilt the buttocks toward the ceiling, hollowing out the back. Hold for an additional 10 seconds. Repeat three to five times.

It is also important that the athlete understand the concepts of core strengthening, which will be further detailed in Chapter 9.

## DISC HERNIATIONS OF THE LUMBAR SPINE

As with the cervical spine, a more severe injury to the lumbar spine is a disc herniation. The most common disc herniations happen at level L4-L5, where the L5 nerve root is pinched, and at level L5-S1, where the S1 nerve root is pinched.

An L5 nerve impingement causes weakness extending all the way to the big toe, and can cause numbness and pain on the top of the foot and pain in the buttocks. An S1 nerve impingement causes ankle reflex and weakness during ankle push-off when running and walking. Numbness and radiating pain may extend all the way down to the bottom of the foot, as well as into the associated muscles.

### Treatment of Disc Herniations of the Lumbar Spine

As with any disc herniation, the athlete should immediately be under the care of both a physician and a physical therapist or athletic trainer to determine a progression of care. The goal is to decrease any present radiculopathy and try to isolate the pain locally to the lumber region. This can be done with RICE, anti-inflammatory medication, and modalities. After radiating symptoms and pain have subsided, the soccer player can start a flexibility and strengthening program to maintain their restored posture.

Herniations can also be treated with sets of exercises designed to resolve any radicular symptoms in the legs and localize pain to the lower back. Once symptoms begin to subside, either of these systems is a great tool for the beginning of rehabilitation. Once flexibility and range of motion have increased, the athlete can begin a core stabilization program, followed by a return to a functional sport routine. Once completing all of these phases in a pain-free manner, the athlete can safely return to play.

Depending on the severity of dysfunction, the physician may elect to administer an epidural, a steroid injection, or even to intervene surgically. It is important to treat any radicular symptoms right away to prevent the long-term effects of nerve-root impingement, such as weakness and disability.

**Prevention of Disc Herniations of the Lumbar Spine**

As mentioned repeatedly in this book, collisions can't be prevented on the soccer field, and these collisions sometimes cause herniated disks. However, if the soccer player is well-conditioned, he or she greatly reduces the risk of injury. The entire body must be trained to endure the demands of the sport. It is important to train both sides of the body equally, utilizing both strength and flexibility components.

# CHAPTER SEVEN

# INJURIES TO THE UPPER EXTREMITIES

Due to the nature of the game, soccer players are usually fairly safe from chronic or overuse injuries to the upper extremities—the shoulder, arm, wrist, and hand—that are seen with overhead sports such as baseball, volleyball, and swimming. However, injuries to the upper extremities can occur, most often as a result of trauma from collision with another player or the turf.

This mechanism tends to result in more severe upper extremity injuries that require a greater amount of time to recover, such as broken bones, dislocations, and subluxations. Signs and symptoms of these injuries are generally more overt, especially in the case of dislocations and displaced broken bones, but this is not always the case. It is possible to have a hairline fracture, in which the fractured bone is nondisplaced and no abnormalities can be observed without advanced imaging.

As long as the integrity of the bone is not at risk, these less severe fractures are often placed in a hard or soft cast for anywhere from three to six weeks to allow adequate time for proper bone healing. These injuries require more judgment on the part of the residing orthopedist, and their orders are dependent on the location of the fracture, the integrity of the bone, evidence of healing, past history, and the age of the athlete. Everything must be taken into account for the doctor to make a decision as to how to manage the athlete, and each case is individual.

If a fracture is suspected during a game or practice, it is important that it is taken care of emergently. Remove the athlete from play, immobilize the area, ice if possible, and seek immediate medical attention.

Fractures generally take six to eight weeks to heal, followed by a four to six week rehab program to return the joint to proper function prior to a return to play. This rehab protocol should be done with a physical therapist or athletic trainer and be supervised by a physician.

## ACROMIOCLAVICULAR JOINT

The shoulder girdle is composed of three bones: the scapula (the shoulder blade, or that bone that looks like a chicken wing on the upper back), the clavicle (collarbone), and the humerus (the long bone in the upper arm) (see Figure 7.1).

The acromioclavicular (AC) joint, also known as the AC joint or shoulder joint, is the junction between the acromion and the clavicle. The acromion process is an extension off of the scapula that articulates with the distal clavicle at the tip of the shoulder. These two bones are held together by three ligaments that extend between them: the AC ligament, the coracoacromial ligament, and the coracoclavicular (CC) ligament (see Figure 7.2). The joint is also stabilized by the coracoid process, which is a hook-like structure that also extends off the scapula. Although these ligaments of the AC joint are very strong, they are vulnerable to traumatic injury because of their location and the small space they occupy.

The AC joint, and the head of the humerus directly below, make up the ball-and socket joint of the shoulder. The freedom of motion allowed at this joint is necessary for functionality in our daily lives and is especially important to athletic activity. However, it is also important to maintain a level of stability within the joint to ensure the integrity of the joint and prevent injury. Balance between mobility and functional stability is key; the

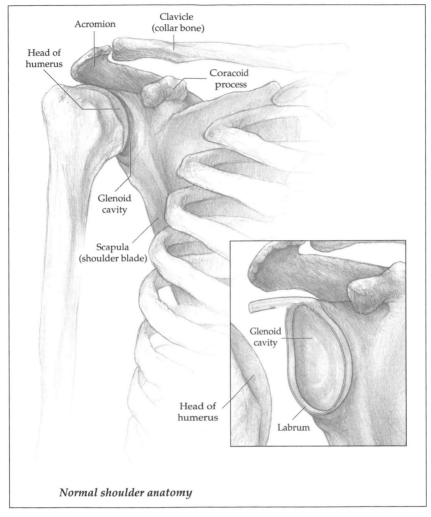

*Normal shoulder anatomy*

**Figure 7.1** Anatomy: Bones of the shoulder girdle.

*Source*: Image reprinted with permission from *Sports Medicine: Study Guide and Review for Boards*, by Mark Harrast and Jonathan Finnoff, Demos Medical Publishing, 2011.

shoulder joint must be lax enough to allow free range of motion, but stable enough to prevent subluxations.

## Mechanism of Subluxation of the Acromioclavicular Joint

When a shoulder subluxation, or separation, is diagnosed, it is important to identify the mechanism of injury so the practitioner has a good idea of what structures have potentially been

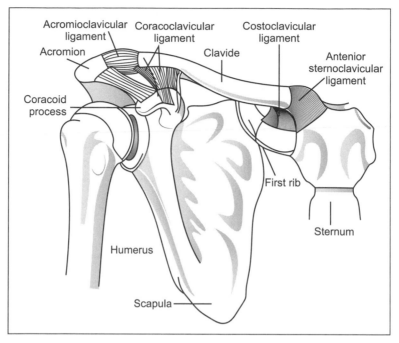

**Figure 7.2** Anatomy: Acromioclavicular ligaments.

damaged or stressed. When shoulder subluxations occur in soccer, they are usually caused by a direct blow to the tip of the shoulder, or from a fall on an outstretched hand.

There are six classifications of an AC separation, ranging in severity from type 1 through type 6. In soccer medicine, our focus is on types 1 through 3, as anything beyond this level requires surgical intervention followed by a rehabilitation protocol detailed by an orthopedic surgeon.

### Classifications of AC Joint Separation

**Type 1**: This injury is basically like spraining a ligament. It is a partial tear of the AC ligament only, with no injury to the CC ligament. Symptoms are point tenderness, mild swelling, and painful range of motion. With appropriate acute care management, the athlete can return to play with no problems, sometimes wearing a donut-like dispersive pad around the AC joint.

**Type 2**: This injury involves both the AC ligament and the CC ligament. It will cause the joint to look as if it has a mild step deformity, where the clavicle is raised higher than the acromion. All motions will be severely painful, but especially shoulder flexion and horizontal adduction, given the degree to which these two motions pinch down the space between the AC joint. This injury must be evaluated by a physician and requires long-term rehabilitation with an athletic trainer or physical therapist.

**Type 3**: This injury includes a complete tear of the AC and CC ligaments. The AC joint appears totally abnormal, with severe swelling and a definitive step deformity. There will be extreme pain and tenderness throughout the entire area. This injury must be evaluated by a physician and can take up to six weeks to properly rehabilitate with an athletic trainer or physical therapist.

### On-Field Evaluation of AC Joint Subluxation

Shoulder subluxations are almost always the result of a forceful collision between the tip of the shoulder and another object, such as a baseball player running into the outfield wall, a quarterback being sacked with his arms held at his side or a soccer player coming down onto the turf after a header. When this injury is sustained on the field, it is good to immobilize by keeping the athlete's arm close to his or her body in a sling position. If a sling is available, this will further help to let the arm rest and take pressure directly off the injury site. Ice is great for the management of pain and inflammation. An orthopedic evaluation is necessary to determine the extent of the injury, as well as to rule out any fractures.

### Rehabilitation of a Subluxated AC Joint

The initial goal of therapy is to decrease pain and inflammation while assisting the body to heal naturally. Following this stage is a progression to a normal shoulder range of motion (see Figures 7.3–7.6). Until there has been adequate time for healing of the ligament, any motions that will open up the joint and stress the damaged ligaments should be avoided. This includes anything where the arm is brought overhead or across the body. With this in mind, the athlete should use the opposite arm for all daily activities; that is, brushing teeth, combing hair, and putting on a shirt properly (using the bad arm first, then the head, then the good arm).

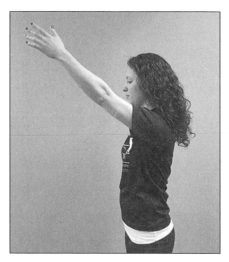

**Figure 7.3** Shoulder flexion: Using the shoulder muscles and keeping the arm straight, elevate the arm in front of you, and elevate it over your head.

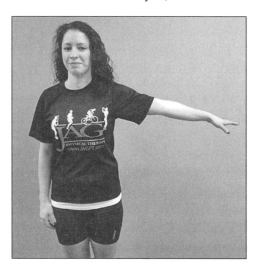

**Figure 7.4** Shoulder abduction: Using the shoulder muscles and keeping the arm straight, raise the arm out to the side, and extend it upward over your head, in the frontal plane.

Based on the level of swelling and bruising, the way the patient carries his or her arm, and the description of symptoms, the treating therapist will determine when there has been adequate time for healing. The athlete can then begin with passive movements, such as pendulum swings. This is a good way to use gravity to assist movement, and will deactivate the surrounding musculature that can often cause pain with motion.

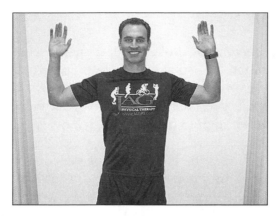

**Figure 7.5** Shoulder external rotation: An outward rotation of the humerus within the ball-and-socket joint of the shoulder.

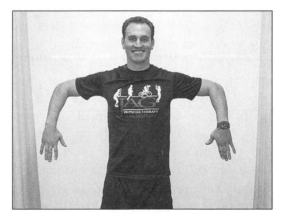

**Figure 7.6** Shoulder internal rotation: An inward rotation of the humerus within the ball-and-socket joint of the shoulder.

A good progression for range of motion exercises goes from passive, to active-assisted, to active range of motion. With an AC separation in particular, it is less stressful to first perform motions with the arm at the patient's side, then to progress to flexion and abduction.

After range of motion is restored with minimal pain, the athlete can start a shoulder strengthening program, which should include flexion/extension, abduction/adduction, horizontal abduction/horizontal adduction, and internal/external rotation exercises. Since the shoulder is a dynamic joint that moves freely in all planes of motion, it's important to allow adequate time for rehab prior to returning to play.

## CLAVICULAR FRACTURE

A clavicular fracture, or broken collarbone, is closely related to the AC separation. It also is caused by a forceful impact to the shoulder girdle, or directly to the collar bone. A fall to the turf directly onto the shoulder or onto an outstretched hand can transmit forces enough to fracture this relatively small, but very important bone.

The collar bone is the most superior portion of the shoulder girdle with many muscular attachments that assist in all motions of the shoulder. The most common site of fracture is the distal, or outer, third of the bone, where the shape transitions from concave to convex.

If a broken collarbone is suspected, the athlete needs to see a physician immediately. Usually, this injury can be diagnosed by simply looking at the collarbone, which will have a visible gap or deviation in the bone, but an x-ray is required to truly diagnose the type of fracture and to assess the amount of displacement.

The symptoms include pain that increases with any shoulder motion, swelling, tenderness, bruising, or a bulge near the shoulder. A grinding or crackling sound may also be present with movement, along with stiffness and an inability to move the shoulder away from the body.

The collarbone does not completely harden until the age of 20, which leaves soccer players at the high school, club, or youth sports level open to the most risk of fracture. The collarbone usually heals without any difficulties, but if the fracture is displaced and cannot be corrected with a simple sling, a surgical intervention may be required, and customarily includes a pin or screw to hold the collarbone together while it heals.

Bone healing requires anywhere from six to eight weeks of inactivity to allow the bone to set properly. Once the bone is strong enough for therapy, the physician will prescribe a protocol to restore normal range of motion and baseline strength of the entire shoulder complex. After range of motion and baseline strength are restored, the athlete can progress to a full strength program and return to soccer activities.

When progressing the athlete back to play, it's important to know his or her position. Most soccer athletes don't need much range of motion in their upper body outside of running, pushing off, or sliding. Keep in mind the throw-in, which applies most to midfielders, and the fact that goalies have to repeatedly catch and throw the ball. If a clavicular fracture is sustained by a goalie, there are some soccer-specific drills that must be held back early in rehab; that is, catching the ball over the head, lateral dives onto the shoulder and any throwing motions. It is important to have full clearance by a physician to progress to these activities in the rehab setting, and the athlete should not return to sport until he or she can show the ability to perform these activities in a practice setting.

## THE ROTATOR CUFF

The rotator cuff is a group of muscles around the shoulder that function to stabilize and rotate the shoulder.

As we've discussed, the shoulder girdle is made up of three bones—the scapula, the clavicle, and the humerus. The rotator cuff is a group of four muscles that come together as tendons to connect the scapula to the humerus, including the supraspinatus, subscapularis, teres minor, and infraspinatus. These muscles originate at the scapula, then extend toward and insert at the humerus via their tendons. When we contract or flex these muscles, the teres minor and infraspinatus pull into external rotation, the subscapularis pulls into internal rotation, and the supraspinatus raises the arm.

### Co-Contraction

This term is important to understanding the stability function of the rotator cuff muscles. Internal and external rotation are contrasting actions, and different muscles are responsible for them. Think about this as a game of tug-o-war; when one muscle fires, or contracts, on one side, it pulls in one direction. When another muscle fires on the other side, it pulls in the opposite direction. When they contract on both sides simultaneously, what happens? There's a stalemate, and neither side moves in either direction.

When our internal and external rotators fire simultaneously, or co-contract, there is a dynamic relationship that keeps our humeral head stable within the shoulder socket (see Figure 7.7). This is an important concept in rehabilitation, and is why *rotator-cuff strengthening* is often prescribed in physical therapy.

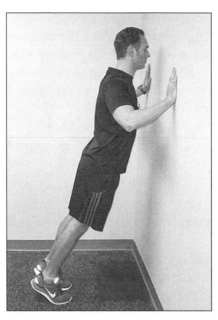

**Figure 7.7** Wall push-up: Place the arms against a wall, directly in front of you at or below shoulder height. Bend the elbows, keeping them at your sides, and press yourself up. This is a good, low-impact way to initiate upper body strengthening.

### Mechanism of Injury to the Rotator Cuff

Rotator cuff tears in soccer are most often suffered by goalies, because, like athletes in swimming, baseball, and tennis, they engage in much more overhead activity.

There are essentially two ways to tear the rotator cuff. The first is the acute tear, suffered when an impact or trauma forces a hyper-rotation of the shoulder. Imagine a goalie falling out to the side on an outstretched arm, and maybe having another player land on top of them. The second is the chronic tear, which is the result of degenerative shearing forces from repetitive action over time; imagine the goalie making the same throw, over and over again.

### Signs and Symptoms of Injuries to the Rotator Cuff

The most common symptoms of rotator cuff tears are pain, weakness, and swelling or stiffness of the shoulder joint. Depending on the extent of the tear and which of the rotator cuff tendons are torn, there will be varying levels of disability. The athlete may even maintain a full range of motion, but will present with weakness in certain directions.

The portion of the rotator cuff most often torn is the supraspinatus, which is used and abused during any overhead throwing activity. This muscle sits on the top of the scapula and runs through a small space between bones before inserting on the humerus. Its function is to elevate the arm (see Figure 7.8), but in doing so, it also gets pinched within the joint space, which makes it prone to degeneration. Of course, there are different predisposing factors, most often postural, that lead to difficulties with this tendon. Any good sports medicine professional can target and correct such problems.

Only an orthopedic surgeon can make a true diagnosis of a rotator cuff tear. The doctor will look for simple signs and symptoms, such as weakness in certain directions of the shoulder. If the doctor suspects a tear, he or she will determine whether or not the soccer player can still do activities without further hurting him- or herself, or if further imaging, such as an x-ray or MRI, is necessary for an accurate diagnosis.

If the injury is determined to be mild, and the athlete is capable of healing on his or her own without surgical intervention, the athlete will be cleared for physical therapy activities and begin a return to sport protocol. As with any other therapy protocol, there will be a progression, beginning with a return to function and the building of foundational strength and mobility, prior to

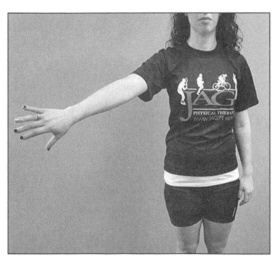

**Figure 7.8** Scaption: Beginning with your arms at your sides, use the shoulder muscles to elevate the arms in front of you, in a Y position at 60 degrees of the frontal plane. Stop at shoulder height.

beginning sport-specific activities. The time frame of return to sport depends on the severity of disability, but in general, a rotator cuff tear in the soccer athlete can be rehabilitated much more quickly than an injury to the lower extremities.

Although the soccer athlete is primarily a running athlete, it's good to include a low-level throwing program prior to returning back to full-go after a rotator cuff tear, especially if the soccer player is a goalkeeper. The goalie should have a good progression of goalie-specific exercises, and should try during the rehabilitative process not to fall on the outstretched arm! This risk should be taken into account and limited by the physical therapist/athletic trainer.

Keep in mind that there are instances where conservative treatment is prescribed in order to avoid surgical intervention. However, if the athlete cannot recover through conservative therapy, surgery may be necessary to repair the rotator cuff. Postsurgical therapy will usually last six months or more, concluding with a full return to sport.

## ULNAR COLLATERAL LIGAMENT

The ulnar collateral ligament (UCL), is a thick, triangular band of tissue on the inner side of the elbow. It connects the distal humerus, or upper arm bone, to the smaller arm bone on the inside of the forearm, the ulna (see Figure 7.9).

The UCL is important in stabilization of the elbow when it is in a slightly flexed position. (When the elbow is in full extension, there is a strong locking mechanism between the bones of the ulna and humerus.) The UCL is composed of an inner and outer portion, known as the anterior and posterior bands.

### Mechanism of UCL Injury

As with most upper extremity injuries, soccer goalkeepers are more likely to suffer a UCL injury than any other player on the field. The UCL can be damaged in either acute or chronic fashion, with the major difference being the mechanism of injury.

In the acute UCL injury, a goalie typically falls on an outstretched arm, often with an external force such as another soccer athlete falling on top of them. A forceful valgus stress is generated at the medial elbow, and an overstretch of the ligament results in a sprain or tear.

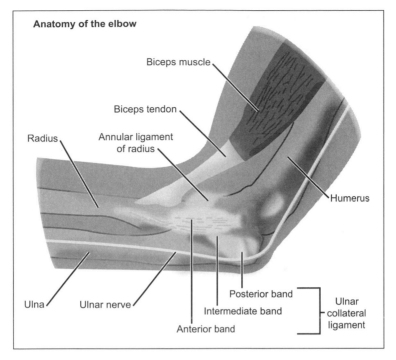

**Figure 7.9** Anatomy of the elbow.

The UCL can also fray like a rope over time. A goalie repeatedly throws the ball in practices and games, which puts stress on the ligament. The stress can eventually cause a laxity in the ligament, which can cause pain and instability.

What's unique about soccer athletes is obviously the size of the ball they're throwing. While a baseball sits nicely in the hand, the circumference and weight of a soccer ball are much greater, so the soccer ball cannot be thrown in the same manner. Try throwing a soccer ball with a bent shoulder and elbow just one time and the inefficiency of the movement will be obvious.

Instead, goalkeepers throw with a straight elbow, utilizing their arm as a long lever and rotating at the trunk. Flexing the wrist around the ball will assist in decreasing the stress at the elbow. This technique can be difficult for the youth athlete, and should be taught early on to all goalkeepers.

It is important to understand that the body works as a biomechanical chain, and to be an efficient thrower, the entire chain must work well. Many young throwing athletes, including goalies, will have poor throwing mechanics and overhead motions; they will often throw only with the shoulder or elbow without utilizing the larger muscle groups in the torso and lower body. As will be discussed in the rehab portion, it is important for every throwing athlete to train the posterior and anterior capsule of the shoulder, maintain good core strength and lower extremity strength, and practice balance and proprioception to utilize the entire kinetic chain when throwing a ball.

### Evaluation of UCL Injuries

If pain in the medial elbow persists over a period of time, the athlete should see a medical professional. A valgus stress test, which opens the medial joint line on the inside of the elbow may be used to assess the integrity of the UCL. An x-ray, ultrasound, or MRI may also be used to further diagnose the injury.

A soccer player can continue to perform at high levels with a grade 1 or mild grade 2 UCL tear. The important thing is to make sure that the athlete will not be at risk for further damage. Protective braces may be used to limit valgus stress at the medial joint line. Taping may also be beneficial.

A grade 3 UCL sprain will require surgical intervention to repair and return the normal structure and function back to the elbow. This surgery is named after Tommy John, the baseball player who first underwent the procedure, and has become very common among baseball players at all levels. Since the UCL has often been completely torn, the surgeon will use an autograft or allograft as an implant to recreate the tensile strength of the ligament and restore integrity to the elbow. The difference between these two grafts is the source: an autograft is from autologous tissue, which is the patient's own, and allologous tissue comes from a cadaver. The physician will choose the type of graph based on both availability and personal preference.

### Treatment of UCL Injuries

Like every other injury we've discussed, UCL injuries can be treated with the RICE protocol and NSAIDs. After pain and swelling subside, the athlete should begin some simple elbow range of motion exercises. Just as we care for the knee and hip when the quadriceps in injured, we must also care for the wrist and shoulder when the elbow is injured, because most muscle groups course the length of multiple joints.

With a UCL sprain, early rehabilitation will consist of light hand and wrist range of motion exercises. The most painful actions are going to be direct elbow flexion/extension and pronation/supination. By initiating range of motion away from the site of injury, we can begin the healing process by activating our skeletal muscle pump (see Figure 7.10). This term describes the influence of skeletal muscle on lymphatic flow, and helps to push inflammation from the extremities back toward the core. Since it is our lymphatic system that is responsible for the distribution and uptake of inflammation, anything we can do to enhance its function is good for business, as long as we're in a pain-free range.

After all elbow, shoulder, wrist, and hand movements are restored to within normal limits, the athlete can begin a good strength program. The progression should start at the wrist with Theraband wrist flexion/extension and supination/pronation exercises, followed by dumbbell resistance exercises. If the athlete can perform those with no pain, he or she can move on to band resistance with elbow flexion and extension, and then on to shoulder resistance exercises. When performing strengthening exercises for the shoulder, be careful about increasing stress at the elbow. Adding a weight in the hand immediately acts as a forceful lever that can stress our medial joint line directly.

Also be careful with the addition of internal and external rotation at the shoulder. These two motions, especially when performed with band or dumbbell resistance, can increase the stress placed on the medial joint line. Before including these motions, make sure there has been adequate healing time, and be sure the shoulder, elbow, and wrist complexes are strong enough to tolerate the added stress.

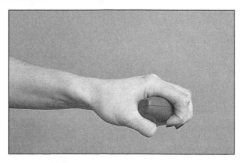

**Figure 7.10** Theraputty squeeze: Using all the fingers individually, and at the same time, squeeze a soft object such as Theraputty, a towel, or a stress ball to increase strength in the forearm, wrist, and hand.

Rehab protocols following UCL repair surgery begin with an immobilization phase with the elbow locked at 90 degrees of flexion with a neutral, upward-pointing thumb. This will allow the graft to set into the bone over the course of the next six to eight weeks. During this time, the patient will follow up with the surgeon and will gradually increase elbow extension in order to minimize the stress put on the new graft. Following this initial postoperative stage, a natural progression into range of motion, strength, neuromuscular control, balance, and proprioceptive exercises can begin (see Figure 7.11). The recovery period following UCL surgery is typically six to nine months, but can be a full year if the patient is predominately a throwing athlete.

**Prevention of UCL Injuries**

In order to prevent UCL injuries, it is important to look at the entire body and the athlete's throwing mechanics. Technically, an athlete generates enough force with each throw to rupture the UCL, but the ligament is protected by muscles and bones that work together to produce motion. This is the kinetic chain, and its sequencing is critical. To throw any ball properly, an athlete must get into the correct position at the correct time

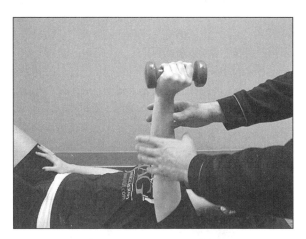

**Figure 7.11** Dynamic shoulder stability: While lying on your back with your arm raised in front of you and a weight in your hand, try to maintain stability while someone tries to knock your arm out of position. This stimulates proprioception and neurological control in the muscles of the shoulder girdle.

with the correct sequence of movements. The instant a thrower's front foot strikes the ground, whether he is a pitcher or a goalie, energy begins to travel up his body. The hips must fully rotate forward, followed by the upper torso, then the shoulders, like dominos falling, before the arm can accelerate to the release point. If the sequencing is out of order, over time the repetitive strain will cause injuries at the weakest link—very often, the elbow. To decrease the incidence of injury to a throwing athlete such as a goalie, all muscle groups must be worked in a properly functioning kinetic chain.

If the athlete is a goalie or other throwing athlete, the posterior aspect of the shoulder is one of the prime places to target to help decrease the incidence of UCL injury. The posterior shoulder is the primary decelerator of the arm during the throwing motion. A good eccentric strengthening program that also addresses the negative component of muscular action is beneficial (see Figure 7.12), along with exercises designed to increase range of motion, specifically with shoulder internal rotation.

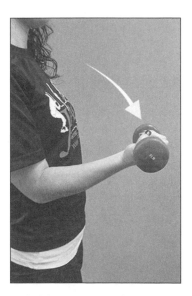

**Figure 7.12** Eccentric biceps strength: With a weight in your hand, begin with your elbow flexed fully toward your shoulder. Focus on the negative as you slowly lower the weight away from your shoulder and down toward your body by extending the elbow.

When looking at commonalities among athletes with shoulder pain and dysfunction, it is well-documented that an individual with an internal rotation deficit has a higher incidence of injury at both the shoulder and elbow. This condition is known as glenohumeral internal rotation deficiency. This exercise can help improve shoulder mobility and increase glenohumeral internal rotation (see Figure 7.13).

## FRACTURES TO THE UPPER EXTREMITY

When an athlete falls on an outstretched hand, there are numerous types of injuries that can occur based on how the athlete lands, such as an elbow dislocation, radial or ulnar head fracture, or metacarpal fracture. Once again, if there is a dislocation or displaced fracture, it can be easy to spot, but if the break in the bone is just a hairline crack, it can present as only wrist or hand pain.

Still, if any type of fracture is suspected, it is important to treat the injury emergently. This may sound obvious, but there are certain types of fractures that may not be so obvious. Parents or coaches should remove the athlete from play, immobilize the area of suspected fracture and RICE! Do not hesitate to activate an emergency medical procedure to alert local EMS of the situation. It's always better to err on the side of caution. In the long term, the athlete should make sure to receive proper care from a physician, which can be directed by an athletic trainer or coach.

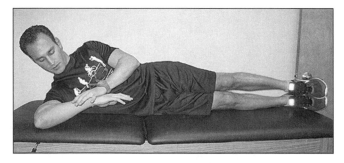

**Figure 7.13** Sleeper stretch: While maintaining a 90-degree angle of shoulder flexion, use the opposite hand to apply downward pressure toward the table, effectively isolating and stretching the posterior shoulder capsule.

## CAN MY SON OR DAUGHTER STILL PLAY WITH A BROKEN BONE IN THEIR HAND OR ARM, OR WHILE WEARING A CAST?

The short answer is yes, but the answer is conditional and hinges on a multitude of factors. An orthopedist must always be the one to decide if a fracture is stable enough for activity. This depends on the severity and location of the fracture, whether or not there was surgery, how much time has been allowed for healing and what position the athlete plays, along with a number of other considerations. Ultimately, the doctor will decide if the risks of returning to play with a cast or brace outweigh the rewards. Keep in mind: it's just a game. The time taken to rest and properly recover is a good investment for the future long-term health of the athlete.

# CHAPTER EIGHT

# CONCUSSIONS

The most common head injury, not only in soccer, but in many other sports today, is the concussion. Parents, coaches, and players all need to recognize that a concussion is not like any other injury. It is a traumatic brain injury that can have lasting effects and can potentially be harmful to daily living by affecting the way we think, feel, and move. Unlike the upper and lower extremities, we have only one brain, and if the brain is injured in any capacity, we can assume cognitive dysfunction on some level will result, with a possible loss of function that can be temporary or permanent.

As the rate of concussions has increased in professional sports and more research has been done about the lasting affects of concussion, the injury has been more and more discussed, both in the medical community and among the general public. Professional sports leagues in the United States have spent millions of dollars investigating the true causes of concussion, along with its lasting effects and treatment, and the treatment of postconcussion syndrome. We have learned that concussions do not only affect the body and how a person physically feels; they can also affect speech, vision, balance, and long- and short-term memory, and can be detrimental to the neurological, psychological, and cognitive well-being of the individual.

With 1.8 million concussions documented yearly in the United States, it is safe to assume that nearly every player, parent, or coach has either experienced concussion first-hand or knows someone who has. And even if they haven't, it is unlikely that any player, parent, or coach has not at least heard about the concussion issue. Its recent relevance in the media has served to alert the public to the dangers of this trauma, and the proper procedural steps to take in the event of injury.

## MECHANISM OF INJURY

A concussion is caused by a trauma to the head, which is any force, either direct or indirect, that brings concussive energy to the brain.

### Direct Trauma

A direct trauma is most obviously caused from a blow to the head that can create enough momentum to cause the brain to slide back and forth against the inner walls of the skull (see Figure 8.1). Although the skull is the brain's primary line of defense against the outside world, the trauma that causes concussion is actually the result of the brain bouncing off of the inside of the skull. Direct trauma can also cause rotational or torsional force of the cranium about its spinal axis. Such rotational forces often result in more severe concussion symptoms.

### Indirect Trauma

Due to the increased knowledge about concussions throughout the world, we have learned that concussions don't only result from direct blows to the head. Concussions are the result of the velocity of the brain within the skull. Any action that causes acceleratory or deceleratory forces can cause a sudden shift of the brain. Imagine a soccer athlete that takes a spill backward and falls on his backside. Force from the hard turf is transmitted up the spine directly to the cranium, providing necessary force to cause concussive trauma. This can be caused by any action that causes a whiplash-like, jerking motion of the head. When these types of motions take place, the brain undergoes immediate biochemical changes. The normal activity of neurotransmitters, the molecules that carry signals from neuron to neuron, is disrupted. Blood flow to the brain is decreased and the ability of neurons to use glucose as fuel is impaired. All of these issues can cause global brain dysfunction.

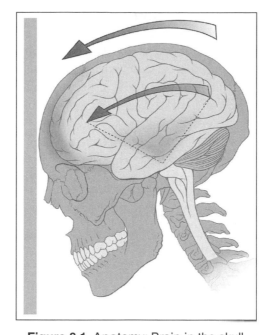

**Figure 8.1** Anatomy: Brain in the skull.

*Source*: Image reprinted courtesy of Patrick J. Lynch, medical illustrator.

## PREVENTION OF CONCUSSIONS

As athletic trainers, we are always of the mindset that the best way to treat an injury is to prevent it altogether. Unfortunately, there are certain assumed risks of participating in sports. Despite these risks, we are always discovering and reinventing our best-practice models to align with the most current research.

As an athletic trainer/physical therapist dealing with soccer players for the last 25 years, I have seen different helmets, padding, and head gear targeted at prevention of concussions. As discussed earlier, concussions are really the result of a trauma to the brain caused by a collision with the inside of the skull. Considering this, we can try using headgear, but in my view, there is really no helmet or additional padding that can act to prevent a concussion.

## SIGNS AND SYMPTOMS OF CONCUSSION

All soccer players, coaches, and parents need to have a general understanding of the common signs and symptoms of a concussion.

Consider the case where two players collide and hit their heads together. On-site medical staff first needs to triage and determine who is most at risk and who needs immediate care. After ruling out a potentially life-threatening injury, the medical staff will go through a checklist and see what's most urgent, keeping in mind there is probably some level of trauma to the brain.

In determining the severity of trauma, medical professionals need to rely on observational data (what can be seen and observed) as well as subjective data (what the athlete is describing). Given that each athlete is an individual, and more so with concussions than any other sports injury, the expressed signs and symptoms are going to vary from person to person.

An important fact to keep in mind is that symptom onset can be immediate, or delayed by days or even weeks. Athletes with potential brain trauma must be evaluated immediately and must continue to be evaluated.

Please note that, contrary to what many people believe, there does *not* need to be a loss of consciousness in order for a concussion to occur. This injury is very specific to the individual, and some people are simply more susceptible than others, with a lower injury threshold.

The most common symptoms of concussion include, but are not limited to, the following:

Headache

Nausea

Vomiting

Dizziness

Fogginess

Confusion

Balance problems

Difficulty concentrating

Other signs and symptoms can vary over time, and can include sensitivity to light, difficulty in concentrating on TV, schoolwork, or conversations, changes in mood, anxiety, depression, sleep disturbances (sleeping more or less), and difficulty sleeping through the night.

As a practitioner, I can tell you that these types of injuries are rarely clear-cut. Signs and symptoms are never the same, they don't always appear right away, and there's no time line on a definitive resolution. We must continue to reevaluate on a daily basis in order to track the progression of symptoms. As stated above, all we truly have is observational and subjective data to rely on. There are also other tools we can use to frame the injury, such as computer programs that define reaction times, memory and delayed recall, but not all athletes will have access to such diagnostic testing.

## TREATMENT

If an athlete is suspected of having a head injury, it is important to have the athlete removed from participation and remain shut down until proper evaluation by a medical professional trained in concussion management can be completed. I cannot stress this enough! If there is even a questionable head trauma, the risks of continued participation are too great to continue playing.

As a health care professional practicing at all levels of competition, I have had the distinct benefit of seeing programs develop over the years and have been able to assess the practicality of various treatment modules.

The best-practice approach, outlined below, is the treatment protocol most accepted within the medical community. It has evolved over the years and is now trickling down from the professional leagues to collegiate and high school athletics.

If concussion symptoms do not resolve within two to three weeks, it may be beneficial to seek the attention of a neuropsychologist for a proper evaluation. Because it may be required later on, it is important to keep good documentation detailing the course of symptoms from the date of injury, as well as any testing done pre- or postinjury.

There are numerous neurocognitive tests available that help extract data that can be useful in diagnosing and defining this tricky injury. For example, the SCAT3 Sport Concussion Assessment Tool is readily downloadable on the Internet for public use, and includes questions that establish cognitive, balance, and coordination baselines for each individual athlete. In the best-practices model, the athlete will take a baseline test such as this one during a preparticipation exam, and will follow with a postinjury exam after symptoms have begun to resolve so the two exams can be compared to assess cognitive function.

When rehabilitating concussions, it is very important that the physician, soccer player, parents, and coaches are all communicating to make sure everyone is on the same page and there are clearly defined objectives.

After symptoms have resolved and the athlete has been cleared by a physician trained in the evaluation and management of concussions, he or she may begin a return-to-play protocol under the guidance of an athletic trainer or physical therapist. This physical return-to-play protocol consists of six stages, and each stage must be successfully completed in succession in order to return to play. Successful completion of a stage is defined by going through the defined protocol asymptomatically.

## PHYSICAL POSTCONCUSSION RETURN-TO-PLAY PROTOCOL

**Stage 1:** No activity. Physical and cognitive rest. Minimum one week removal from all exertional activities. Possible removal from school. After a full week of being symptom-free, progress to stage 2.

*Objective:* Allow for a complete resolution of symptoms prior to introducing physical or cognitive stress that may exacerbate symptoms.

**Stage 2:** Introduction of light aerobic exercise, at less than 70% of maximum heart rate, on an arc trainer, stationary bike, or elliptical machine. Conditioning must be low-impact conditioning to prevent jarring to the cranium. Duration should be between 20 and 40 minutes, depending on the athlete's prior conditioning level, which is dependent on the athlete's sport and activity level.

*Objective:* Introduction of mild aerobic stress. Often, when returning from concussion, symptoms may emerge with an increase in blood pressure. The residing athletic trainer or physical therapist will monitor the program and evaluate the athlete's progress. *Note:* Max heart rate is calculated using the formula 220–age. Multiply this by 0.70 to get the target of 70%. Example: 70% of maximum heart rate for a 15-year-old athlete is 140 bpm.

**Stage 3:** Introduction of low-impact activities. Begin with a warm-up on the bike or elliptical and progress to body-weight exercises like lunges and squats, then to a light jog. Introduce light shuffling, cutting, and ladder drills.

*Objective:* Maintain the same level of intensity as stage 2, but increase the length of time exercising to 20 to 60 minutes, mimicking the demands of the athlete's sport.

**Stage 4:** Incorporation of noncontact, sport-specific drills. Conditioning intensity can increase to include sprinting, running, and cutting drills. Progressive resistive exercises with stretch bands and strength bands can also be introduced.

*Objective:* To continue to be symptom-free as activity level increases. Upon successful completion, the athlete should be reevaluated by a physician trained in the management of concussions.

**Stage 5:** Return to practice. Day 1 at 50%, participating in half of the reps as the rest of the team. No contact or collision. The athlete can progress to a full practice as long as symptoms do not recur. Continue with cardio and strength training. The athlete must achieve his or her prior level of conditioning before returning to any soccer game.

*Objective:* To stress the athlete in as close to full-participation as possible without the risk of reinjury or the return of symptoms.

**Stage 6:** Symptom-free. The athlete is basically back to normal. Full medical clearance from a physician trained in the management of concussions is given. The athlete can then participate in a full-contact soccer practice.

*Objective:* Establish acclimatization back into their team sport. This stage is necessary, mostly as a confidence builder, and must be achieved before a soccer player can reenter the game.

Returning to sport postconcussion is a delicate process. This is a vague injury, with various symptoms that may or may not be present, and that may develop over time. Since there is such an open-ended description of details, there is just as open-ended a return-to-play protocol. There is much room for interpretation, and even creativity, on the practitioner's part. As general objectives are defined, guidelines are followed, and common sense is practiced, the athlete can have a safe and healthy return to sport.

Athletes, parents, and coaches are often frustrated by the lengthiness of the return-to-sport protocol following concussion, and sometimes feel medical professionals are being over-bearing or too careful. This may be true, but the risks involved are too great to ignore, and due to the potentially damaging effects of concussion, it is much safer to err on the side of caution. Further, this protocol allows for a logical, graded progression back into sport. All is evidence-based, and the goal of the medical professional is to safely prepare and return the athlete back to the field. Of course, if an athlete does not adequately complete a stage of rehabilitation, he or she may be held back, but the converse is also true. If the athlete hits the benchmarks earlier, he or she can move more quickly through the program.

## RETURN TO COGNITION

In addition to reacquiring the physical skills and conditioning needed for a return to sport, the athlete must also recover cognitively. For the student–athlete, it is important to include teachers and guidance counselors in the conversation so the necessary accommodations can be made. The athlete should be aware that any cognitive stressors may delay recovery and/or exacerbate symptoms. These include reading, television, video games, and texting. All of these things require brain function (at least on some level!). So don't forget, though mild, a concussion is a *brain injury*.

The stages of cognitive return to function include modifications for gradual reintegration into a full day of class or work. Similar to our physical return-to-play protocol, each stage needs to be completed in succession. If during any stage the soccer player exhibits any return of concussion symptoms, or the onset of new symptoms, he or she should be pulled back from the current level of cognitive activity. Following 24 hours of rest, the athlete may continue to progress through the program.

Based on new concussion research, an overwhelming majority of states have actually passed legislation on concussion safety that details proper treatment protocols. Those that have not yet passed legislation are in the process of doing so.

## STAGES FOR COGNITIVE RETURN TO FUNCTION

| STAGE | ACTIVITY | OBJECTIVE |
|---|---|---|
| No activity | Complete cognitive rest—no school, homework, reading, texting, video games, or computer | Recovery and resolution of symptoms |
| Gradual reintroduction of cognitive activity | Add back above restrictions for short periods of time; 5–15 min | Gradual increase in subsymptom threshold cognitive activities |
| Homework at home before school work at school | Homework in longer increments (20–30 min at a time) | Increase cognitive stamina by repetition of short periods of cognitive activity |
| School reentry | Part day of school after tolerating 1–2 cumulative hours of homework at home | Reentry into school with accommodations |
| Gradual reintegration into school | Increase to full day of school | Accommodations decrease as cognitive stamina improves |
| Resumption of full cognitive workload | Introduce testing, catch up with essential work | Full return to school; may commence return-to-play protocols |

*Source*: The Buffalo Concussion Clinic

## RECURRENT CONCUSSIONS

It is important to note that repeated concussions may lower an athlete's "concussion threshold." That is, the force of impact required to produce concussion symptoms will be lower than it was prior to the athlete's first concussion. Repeated concussions can also lead to more severe and longer-lasting symptoms with each successive injury. This is why it is important to know how many concussions an athlete has had over the course of his or her season or career. As a general rule, any athlete who suffers three concussions in one season should be done for the season, and should be examined by a neurologist.

### What Is Chronic Traumatic Encephalopathy?

Recent headlines have featured more and more retired athletes from the NFL with troubling outcomes following successful careers. It is believed by most medical professionals that through years of traumatic abuse to the brain due to the rigors of their sport, a build-up of tau protein develops around brain tissue, causing a condition called chronic traumatic encephalopathy (CTE). This protein has chemical effect on the brain and negatively affects its function. Up until recently, accurate diagnosis could only be obtained through an autopsy. However, recent developments in MRI have been able to detect the presence of this protein in living patients.

CTE is certainly not exclusive to retired NFL players. This has also been seen historically in boxing, and is often described as being "punch-drunk." Symptoms include chronic headaches, depression, difficulty concentrating, memory problems, personality and emotional changes, parkinsonism, and even early onset Alzheimer's disease. CTE has also been found in military veterans coming back from battle who have had exposure to concussive forces. As it is currently understood, CTE develops after years of repeated, subconcussive forces. That is, forces that jar the brain but are not necessarily significant enough to cause a concussion.

Any athlete that suffers repeated head trauma could subsequently suffer from CTE. It is therefore very important for athletes, coaches, and parents to understand the severity of concussions and to treat them seriously and conservatively. Even mild concussive symptoms should be reported for proper evaluation by a medical professional.

# CHAPTER NINE

# STRENGTH AND CONDITIONING

When athletes define their fitness goals, they must take into account what attributes are desirable for their chosen sport. Soccer athletes don't train the same way as power lifters, who don't train the same way as swimmers. So, what abilities or traits give the ideal soccer player success on the field? Speed, quickness, agility, flexibility, strength, stamina, and balance. Soccer athletes must include a good strength and conditioning program to improve these attributes across the board. The program should target the athlete's weaknesses in an effort to improve upon them.

The same strength and conditioning attributes that make the athlete a better soccer player also serve to keep him or her strong, healthy, and injury-free. If time is invested in strength and conditioning on a daily basis, many injuries can be prevented, especially over the course of a long season when the body needs to be in peak condition. Our goal as fitness professionals is to improve the athlete's foundational fitness attributes away from the field, through a logical strength and conditioning program.

Of course, good soccer players also have incredible, sport-specific skills, such as touch and striking ability on the ball.

No amount of time in the gym will prepare an athlete for what happens on the field; to get better at soccer, we need to get outside and play it!

Though fitness is always a goal for athletes, it is equally important for the athlete to compete on a regular basis. Competition is the force that drives us to better ourselves, and to hone our skills over the course of time.

The objective of this chapter is to provide the athlete with a framework for a good strength and conditioning program so the athlete can design and implement an individualized program. It is important to organize the program in a logical progression that will lay the foundation for success in soccer. The reason for such a generalized approach is that there is no single program that can give you the speed, strength, and ability that will guarantee success in soccer. However, it is important to be knowledgeable in your approach to strength and conditioning, and to understand planning and goal setting as it relates to a strength and conditioning program.

## ENERGY SYSTEMS

What fuels an athlete? There are three energy systems, or bioenergetics, that overlap and work together on a cellular level to physiologically produce energy and effectively fuel our bodies during activity (see Figure 9.1). Two of the systems, the phosphagen and glycolytic systems, are anaerobic systems, which run in the absence of oxygen. The third system, the aerobic system, operates in the presence of oxygen. All of these run on different time frames, offering varying intensity levels lasting from several seconds to several hours.

### Anaerobic Systems

Anaerobic systems are fueled by currently available energy molecules present in our skeletal muscle, known as adenosine triphosphate (ATP). ATP is used during exercise and takes time to replenish, and can only be replenished in the presence of oxygen. In the short term, there is a limited supply. Thus, when the body is operating anaerobically, rapid exhaustion will result from the limited supply of energy molecules.

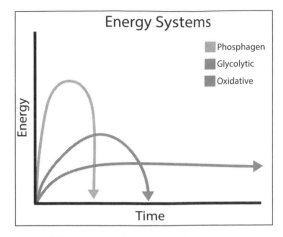

**Figure 9.1** Energy system graph.

### The Phosphagen System

During short-term, intense bursts of exercise, a large amount of power needs to be produced by the muscles, which creates a huge demand for ATP. The phosphagen system is the quickest synthesizer of ATP. Because this system runs in the absence of oxygen, and the body relies on oxygen for nearly everything it does, and because the body has a limited supply of ATP molecules, we cannot last very long within this system. Exercise fueled by the phosphagen system only lasts about 10 seconds before exhaustion. This type of exercise is of high intensity, and requires a maximal effort. Example exercises include single rep max-effort power lifts and meter sprints.

### The Glycolytic System

This system is in the mid-range and lies between the phosphagen and aerobic systems. It is the second-fastest synthesizer of ATP; during this phase, blood glucose is broken down and usable ATP is produced. Exercise fueled by this system lasts in the 30-second to two-minute range before exhaustion. Example exercises include 100-meter sprints with time allowed for recovery.

### The Aerobic System

The aerobic system is the most complex of the three energy systems. It is run in the presence of oxygen; "aerobic" means "requiring air." While this system produces the most ATP, it is also the slowest synthesizer of ATP. This means the aerobic system can't fuel exercise that requires the fast production of ATP, but at a steadier pace, its capacity is virtually inexhaustible. This is the body's primary energy system; it is constantly churning and is responsible for replenishing the other two systems. Aerobic exercises are of long duration and low intensity. Examples include long-distance running, biking, or swimming.

It is important to remember that these energy systems are not independent of one another. They all work and run simultaneously during activity. However, depending on the specific demands placed on an athlete, one energy system may be taxed more than the others over the course of a practice, game, or training session. It is therefore important to stress each system on a weekly and even daily basis in training in order to be ready for every type of athletic situation. Please note that since the aerobic system is always churning, it is possible to increase aerobic capacity in an anaerobic training environment. For example, both a five-mile run and multiple 100-meter sprints will increase aerobic capacity.

## THE PHYSICAL DEMANDS OF SOCCER

Soccer athletes typically run for 90-plus minutes per match, and generally rely on the long-term endurance provided by their aerobic systems more than the other bioenergetics systems. Of course, throughout the course of match play, there will also be shorter, intermittent sprints that tax the anaerobic systems.

Fitness must be improved in all systems in order for the athlete to make overall gains. Training regimens must be varied to incorporate the different phases and expected demands of soccer. Through constant variation, athletes can prepare their bodies for any unknown challenge that is thrown their way.

Soccer athletes must be fit for soccer. That fitness includes overall health. The fittest athlete is not only the one who is able to compete at the highest level, but also the one who is able to compete in the most competitions over the course of a long season. Losing time to injury is often unavoidable, but athletes can limit their time away from the field by taking care of their bodies as much as possible.

## TARGET TRAINING ZONES

Athletes should target themselves between 60% and 85% of their maximum heart rate through the course of their training. Various studies have shown that athletes training in this range, from 30 to 45 minutes per day, are truly working at an aerobic threshold, which will improve their endurance, lung capacity, and general fitness. As stated earlier, it is equally beneficial to train for shorter durations at higher intensities, stressing the various energy pathways in preparation for sport.

A simple formula can be used to determine an athlete's maximum heart rate. By subtracting the athletes age from 220, we get an estimated maximum heart rate. For example, a 15-year-old athlete will have an estimated maximum heart rate of 205 beats per minute (bpm). From this number, we can calculate our percentages; that is, 60% is 0.60 × 205, or 123 beats per minute.

Athletes can take their pulse to check their heart rate during activity, either at the inside of the wrist or at the carotid artery at the side of the neck (see Figure 9.2). Count the number of beats in 15 seconds, and multiply by four. If that's too difficult, just count out the entire minute!

Outside of this guideline, athletes should train within their means with respect to their age to prevent risk of injury.

As athletes train and become more and more physically fit, they will ultimately see an improvement, or a decrease, in their resting heart rates. As determined by the American Heart Association, the resting heart rate of the average individual should be between 60 and 80 beats per minute. However, elite athletes can fall as low as 35 to 50 beats per minute.

### Anaerobic Training

Hardcore, high-level athletic training usually falls somewhere between 80% and 90% of an athlete's maximum heart rate. This is the anaerobic training zone. This type of activity is done in short bursts, from just seconds all the way up to about

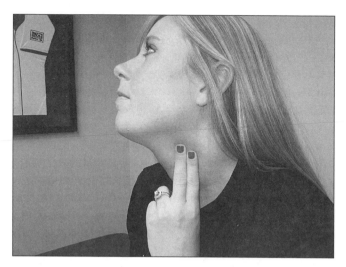

**Figure 9.2** Carotid pulse: Using your left or right pointer and middle fingers, locate the carotid artery on the same side of the neck, just below the angle of the jaw. The carotid pulse is very strong and should be easily felt. Do not use your thumb because it has a pulse of its own.

two minutes. In the absence of oxygen, high-intensity exercise will cause lactic acid to form quickly in the muscles. This type of training is used to promote strength. It is important to train in this zone to help build muscle mass and improve speed and explosiveness.

Example exercises include short sprints, hills, and explosive jumps that will build the overall body strength that is crucial to an athlete in the 70th minute of a match when the muscles are thoroughly fatigued.

### Aerobic Training

The soccer athlete runs an average of six to seven miles in any given match. In order to handle that much running, the aerobic fitness of soccer players needs to be at peak levels. Aerobic training should be done at around 60% to 75% of maximum heart rate. As stated earlier, the aerobic system is constantly running to produce energy and replenish lost energy stores within our muscles. Improving the body's ability to generate and regenerate lost energy stores will improve the body's capacity to reduce lactic acid build-up in the muscles, and will subsequently increase strength and conditioning.

It is my recommendation that athletes should be in the gym or weight room two to three times per week in season and three to four times per week out of season. In-season training is necessary to maintain strength levels throughout the course of a rigorous season, without overtaxing the body. Offseason training should be programmed to improve overall strength and conditioning levels across all competencies; this is when the biggest gains are made.

Make sure off days are scheduled into every strength and conditioning program; the body benefits just as much from rest as it does from work.

My recommendation is to do a full-body strength routine with three sets of 10 reps. As the soccer athlete progresses into more formalized programs, strength and conditioning becomes a truly integral part of his or her training. Licensed strength coaches will teach different levels of rest, periodization, pyramid systems, and various other techniques and programming. For the purposes of the young athlete, the larger muscle groups should be broken down: quads, hamstrings, calves, chest, upper back, shoulders, and arms. Some recommended exercises are squats, calf raises, dumbbell rows and raises, pushups, and bicep curls.

Remember, always have a partner or spotter, even when training at home in the basement. Be sure to get full range of motion in the entire joint for maximum benefit; range of motion is the distance a lever can move while attached to a fixed point. Imagine your bones as levers and the joints as fixed points, and make sure you exercise them from full flexion to full extension.

### Core Training

The core is a very important part of any athlete. But what exactly is it? It's basically the torso; the body minus the arms and legs. The core includes all the muscles of the abdomen, the lower back, and the upper hip. These muscles are necessary for continual spinal stabilization and rotational stability. When the core is strong and stable, many injuries can be prevented. Exercises to improve core strength are not limited to standard flexion or crunch abdominal exercises, but must also incorporate an extension component. Examples include the superman, done on all fours while raising the arms and legs off of the ground. This is a great way to incorporate the back side of the body and maintain balance in the front and back, as well as on both sides (see Figures 9.3–9.5).

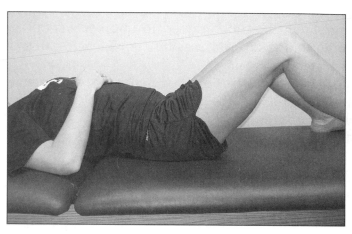

**Figure 9.3** Pelvic tilt: In a supine position with the feet planted and knees elevated, contract the abdomen, keeping the spine stable. Simultaneously rotate the pelvis by arching your back, and then rotate the opposite direction by forwardly rotating your hips. The feet, buttocks, and shoulders should always be in contact with the ground.

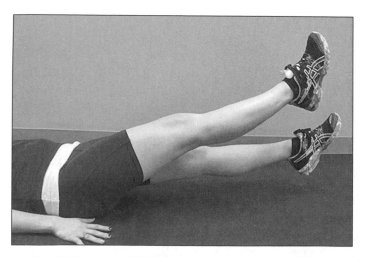

**Figure 9.4** Flutter kicks: While keeping a tight core and straight legs, elevate the feet six inches off the ground and alternate raising and lowering your legs. Your feet should never touch the ground. Complete sets of 30 seconds each.

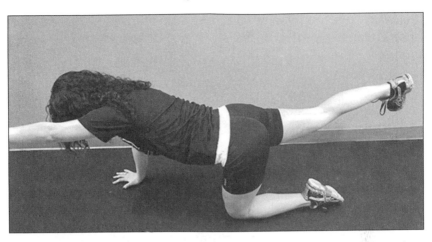

**Figure 9.5** Alternating quadruped superman: While in a quadruped position on all fours, simultaneously extend the right arm and left leg while maintaining a tight core and square hips. Hold for three seconds. Repeat on the opposite side. Do 10 repetitions.

## FLEXIBILITY

Flexibility is a simple and extremely necessary component of every strength and conditioning program. Training causes fatigue in the muscles, which can cause them to tighten. Spasms in tight muscles can cause pain. Too much training can result in over-use injuries. Running athletes are most commonly sore with tight hamstrings and external rotators such as the piriformis and glutes. Soreness from training can make everyday activities difficult to perform, but with adequate flexibility, the activities of daily living are easy.

Flexibility is also a key part of most rehabilitation protocols and is always essential to the prevention of athletic injury.

There are two primary ways athletes can improve their flexibility through standard techniques. In *static stretching*, muscles are elongated into a static stretch that is typically held for a period of 30 seconds. The stretch is usually repeated three times. Though this technique has value and should be included in strength and conditioning programs, *ballistic stretching* has more benefits than static stretching. Ballistic stretching is a technique that utilizes a rapid elongation of the muscle followed by a rapid shortening. Examples of ballistic stretches are high-knees, squat jumps, and side-shuffles. This manner of stretching is proven to increase blood flow deep within the muscles, increasing the body temperature and the flexibility of the skeletal muscle.

A good warm-up or cool-down should include both static and ballistic stretching components that target the specific muscles used repeatedly in soccer. Soccer athletes must engage in all sorts of dynamic motion; forward running, backward running, diagonal running, jumping, kicking, passing, and rotating. All of these different mechanical motions require different demands at each limb, directed through the torso. It is important to keep these various and specific actions in mind when designing a stretching protocol and strength and conditioning program, as well as when rehabilitating an injury.

I recommend that every athlete does some sort of flexibility workout every day. Preactivity, stretches should be done after a 10- to 15-minute warm-up during which the athlete has broken a sweat. Postactivity, stretches should be held for 20 to 30 seconds and should address all muscles used during activity, including the quadriceps, hamstrings, piriformis, calves, hip flexors, abdominals, lower back, groin and adductors, iliotibial band, and shoulders.

# CHAPTER TEN

# HYDRATION AND NUTRITION

Athletes often forget that injuries can be prevented through proper nutrition and hydration. Yes! If athletes eat and drink to properly fuel their bodies, they will stay healthier!

Soccer athletes should have a good understanding of what it means to fuel their body in preparation for the physical demands of their sport, as well as what foods to stay away from.

We already know that a soccer player covers six to seven miles in any given match. Of course, youth athletes will cover less ground, but will still run about three miles per game. Regardless of level, soccer athletes are in constant motion and their bodies must be properly fueled to handle that amount of exercise.

## HYDRATION

Hydrate or die. That's the truth. In soccer, the ramifications of improper hydration may not always be so severe, but they can still lead to injuries, fatigue, and cramping. Soccer athletes must understand what it means to be properly hydrated, when to hydrate, and how hydration aids in injury prevention.

Sixty percent of our entire body mass and 90 percent of our blood is made up of water! Our bodies crave water, and we have to give our bodies what they want, especially during intense training and activity. Physiologically, water assists the human body in almost every function. It keeps the vital organs working properly, lubricates the joints, maintains blood viscosity, prevents muscle fatigue and cramps, and is a major contributor to skin-cooling, which keeps the core body temperature at an optimal level.

Athletes lose two to three liters (L) of water per hour during exercise. To ensure optimal performance, and to maintain overall health, that water must be replenished. Water should not be used by parents or coaches as a reward or goal. It should not be withheld until a certain number of sprints have been finished, or as punishment for poor performance. As parents and coaches, we need to educate our children about the benefits of hydration as well as about warning signs of dehydration. Just as it's important for youth athletes to learn soccer drills and skills, it's crucial for them to understand how the body works and how to take care of it. Water should be readily available during all athletic activity, and water breaks should be programmed into all practice schedules, especially if the environment is high-risk.

### How to Hydrate

Coaches, parents, and athletic trainers should encourage their athletes to prehydrate prior to activity. This process begins about 72 hours in advance of competition, but hydration should be thought of as a good maintenance practice to include in the daily routine. The Food and Drug Administration (FDA) recommends drinking six to eight, 8-ounce glasses of water per day for a normal healthy lifestyle. This recommendation is universal, and is a good practice to keep the body in peak physical condition.

During activity, athletes should rehydrate with 6 ounces of fluid every 15 minutes. Sports drinks are fine, but keep in mind that most sports drinks contain large amounts of sugar that are not necessary to the hydration process. In a very hot or humid setting, too much sports drink can cause nausea, bloating, and diarrhea. Water is usually sufficient for hydration.

**REMEMBER: IF YOU'RE THIRSTY, IT'S TOO LATE!**

**Prehydrate:** Begin 72 hours in advance of competition

**Hydrate During Activity:** Six ounces every 15 minutes

**Rehydrate:** Drink 32 ounces of liquid per 1 pound of fluid loss

## WHAT IS A *"HIGH-RISK ENVIRONMENT?"*

A high-risk environment is one in which external conditions increase an athlete's chances for heat-related illness by inhibiting the body's ability to cool itself. How does the body cool itself during activity? With sweat! The main function of sweat is to keep the core body temperature down through a process known as *evaporative cooling*. It may sound complex, but it is actually quite intuitive. When our body temperature rises during activity, it elevates from the core and disperses out through the skin. As sweat evaporates, it provides a cooling mechanism that draws heat away from the body. When this mechanism is functioning normally, as it does in most healthy individuals, it protects us from heat-related illnesses.

Abnormal functioning of the body's evaporative cooling system can cause the core body temperature to rise to potentially fatal levels. Some risk factors that can cause the body's evaporative cooling system to malfunction can be controlled, while others cannot. We need to take care of the ones we can control, and properly manage the ones we cannot. As coaches, players, and parents, we need to be aware of the dangers, and manage the risk factors that elevate the chances of heat-related illness.

## INTERNAL RISK FACTORS FOR HEAT-RELATED ILLNESS

- **Dehydration:** This is the first warning sign of potential heat illness. *Rule of thumb:* If you're thirsty, it's too late! Since our blood is 90% water, lower water volume will cause the blood to become thick and viscous, which makes it more difficult for the heart to pump blood to the muscles and organs.

- **High body mass index (BMI):** Athletes who are overweight or have a higher BMI will have a more difficult time cooling themselves, because the excess fat traps heat inside the body. While these charts do not take into account lean muscle mass, they are a quick and easy way to get a general idea of what a proper BMI range should be.
- **Improper acclimatization:** It takes the body anywhere from 3 to 14 days to be properly acclimatized to a new environment. It is important for coaches to realize that athletes will not be able to perform as well, and are at a higher risk for heat illness in the first days of practice, when the body may still be adjusting to climate change.
- **Heart disease:** If an athlete is known to have a heart condition prior to activity, he or she must analyze the risks of putting the heart under the increased stresses created by physical activity. This is generally determined by a physician during a preparticipation exam, and overseen by an athletic trainer, coach, or parent.
- **Hypertension:** High blood pressure forces the heart to pump harder and faster. During physical activity, the heart is already under extra stress, and heat and improper hydration can increase that stress.

## EXTERNAL RISK FACTORS FOR HEAT-RELATED ILLNESS

- **High heat index:** The heat index combines air temperature with relative humidity to determine an apparent temperature; that is, how hot does it actually feel? (see Figure 10.1).
- **Humid air:** When there is excessive moisture in the air, it prohibits the evaporation of moisture from the skin, which inhibits the body's evaporative cooling process.
- **Saturated clothing:** Saturated clothing against the skin also prohibits the evaporation of moisture from the skin, which inhibits the body's evaporative cooling process.

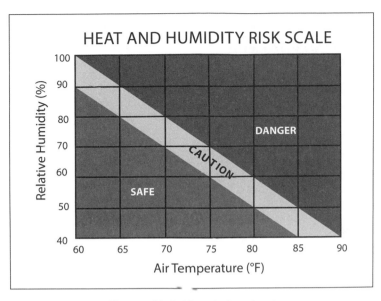

**Figure 10.1** Heat index chart.

## SIGNS AND SYMPTOMS OF HEAT-RELATED ILLNESS

There are three main types of heat illness: heat cramps, heat exhaustion, and heat syncope (also known as heat stroke), which is fainting as a result of heat-related illness. All are brought about with exertion, generally with unsafe environmental stressors as contributing factors. Each condition varies in severity, and they usually occur in succession from one to the next.

As mentioned above, physical exertion in a high-risk environment will decrease the body's ability to thermo-regulate via evaporative cooling. Even with proper hydration, continuing to physically stress the body in a risky environment is potentially hazardous. This is essentially the mechanism of injury when looking at heat illness, which can be intensified with multiple risk factors. Listed in the chart on the following page are some common signs and symptoms of each heat-related illness, and what to do if they occur.

### Heat Cramps

Heat cramps are an early-warning sign that a heat stress is developing. They most often occur in the lower extremities.

| ILLNESS | SIGNS AND SYMPTOMS | TREATMENT |
|---------|--------------------|-----------|
| Heat cramps | Involuntary muscle contraction | Remove from play<br>Put muscle on stretch for immediate relief<br>Rehydration |
| Heat exhaustion | Redness of skin<br>Profuse sweating<br>Nausea<br>Vomiting | Medical emergency<br>Rehydration<br>Ice bags around core (under arms, groin, chest, neck) |
| Heat syncope | Complete inability to thermo-regulate<br>Pale/clammy skin<br>Sweating has ceased<br>Dizziness<br>Nausea<br>Unconsciousness | Medical emergency<br>This individual needs to be rapidly cooled in an ice bath and transported to a trauma center |

Most competitive athletes will try to continue participation, sometimes through rehydrating orally or intravenously where available. However, it is important to stop activity, rest in a cool place, and rehydrate! Sports beverages can help to replenish electrolytes lost through sweat. If cramping does not improve within an hour, seek medical attention. Heat cramps can rapidly accelerate into a life-threatening problem. Furthermore, continuing to play with a cramped muscle can increase the risk of a muscle strain or tear.

**Heat Exhaustion**

At this stage, the soccer player will be experiencing heavy sweating, redness of the skin, and possibly even nausea or vomiting. There can also be symptoms that mimic those of a concussion; headache, blurred vision, dizziness, and possibly fainting. It's important to understand that heat exhaustion is life-threatening! Call 911 immediately. Rapid cooling is crucial. Use of ice baths is recommended if available, and at the very least, saturated clothing should be removed to help bring the core body temperature back to a safe level.

**Heat Syncope, or Heat Stroke**

At this point, the body is completely unable to thermo-regulate, or control its own temperature. The body is no longer producing sweat, the skin is red hot, and the athlete is often in an altered mental state. Fainting is a possibility. Body temperature can be upward of 104° within 10 minutes of identifying a heat illness, and if left untreated, can result in permanent damage to the brain or other vital organs, and possibly even death. Heat stroke kills close to 4,000 Americans per year, so once symptoms are identified, it is important to call 911 immediately and take immediate action to cool the body. This is best achieved with an ice bath, or with ice packs or cold sponges under the armpits and knees and at the groin. Do not give any liquids or solids by mouth.

## NUTRITION

Soccer nutrition must be approached with common sense and an understanding of what it means to properly fuel for competition. I always get a kick out of athletes who can't connect what they're eating during the day with their performance on the field.

Youth and teenage athletes must develop good eating habits that will last them a lifetime. This is the best time to introduce a healthy lifestyle, so they can make the connection between input and output; what we put into our bodies is directly linked to what we get out of our bodies. A bag of chips won't get you through a 90-minute game in the hot afternoon sun. Good nutrition will not only benefit the soccer athlete or the youth athlete; healthy eating habits are important for people of every age and form the foundation for healthy living.

**Macronutrients**

There are three basic macronutrients that make up the basis of our diet: carbohydrates, proteins, and fats. Each macronutrient is essential in its own right, and is a necessary component for a healthy, well-rounded diet. Every meal should include items from each category, whether a person is trying to maintain, lose, or gain weight. Depending on an athlete's nutritional goals, meals may be added or subtracted throughout the day.

A basic guideline is to eat meals consisting of 65% carbohydrate, 20% protein, and 15% fat. Of course, estimations can be made, but the only true way to accomplish this is to weigh our foods.

The soccer player should have a checklist to aid in getting these percentages into their meals and into their bodies. A healthy-eating checklist can include the following:

- Eat breakfast seven days a week
- Eat three to four balanced meals on a regular schedule each day
- Have a nutritious mid-morning snack
- Eat two to three pieces of fresh fruit per day
- Eat four to five servings of fresh vegetables each day (not out of a can!)
- Eat breads or cereals high in fiber
- Eat lean, low-fat proteins (chicken, tuna, steak) at each meal
- Maintain body weight (goal dependent)
- Have a nutritious snack an hour preworkout
- Have a nutritious snack 30 to 45 minutes postworkout
- Eat a well-balanced meal two to three hours before competition
- Hydrate appropriately throughout the day
- Take a daily multivitamin

It is very important that athletes realize proper, consistent nutrition that will help the athlete perform at a high level. It will also help the body heal more quickly, which allows the athlete to consistently participate and stay fit throughout the season. Proper nutrition and hydration can also decrease the risk of muscular injuries, which is what this entire book is about.

### Carbohydrates

Carbohydrates are the first energy source expended by the body during activity. They are easily mobilized and directly available in the bloodstream. Our skeletal muscle needs this quick energy source readily available throughout the course of activity. As we see from marathon runners and their pre-race pasta parties, carbohydrates are necessary to sustain peak levels of performance.

However, if you are not training and burning off carbohydrates as energy, they will eventually be stored as fat. Understand that these guidelines are for athletes training 90 minutes per day, with competitions equally as long. Nonsoccer player guidelines will be slightly different, but only in the amount of intake.

There are three different types of carbohydrates that can be derived from our food choices: slow-, moderate-, and fast-absorbing carbohydrates. Each have their place, and must be included in a well-balanced diet.

### Fast-Absorbing Carbohydrates

Fast-absorbing carbs can be utilized for quick energy almost immediately after consumption. Examples include waffles, pancakes, potatoes, bagels, sport drinks, corn chips, and some fruits, such as watermelon, cantaloupe, and pineapple. These are all high in sugar, and are not always the best choice of carbohydrate. The best times to eat these are prior to athletic activity, and immediately postexercise to replenish lost carbohydrate stores. But be wary, because the body burns these types of carbohydrates so quickly, a "crash" can result if the body is not properly fueled with other foods at regular intervals throughout the day.

### Moderate-Absorbing Carbohydrates

These carbs are the in-between choices that absorb just a little more slowly than those in the fast-absorbing category. Examples include whole-grain breads, high-fiber cereal, brown rice, pasta, oatmeal, sweet potatoes, fruit juice, bananas, grapes, and raisins.

### Slow-Absorbing Carbohydrates

Slow-absorbing carbs are good for long-term dietary maintenance of carbohydrate levels. They are good to include preactivity to increase energy stores for the long-term, so they are readily available when they're needed. Examples include apples, cherries, peaches, plums, pears, chickpeas, milk, yogurt, eggplant, broccoli, and Brussels sprouts.

## Protein

Protein is important for the restoration of muscle fibers following the breakdown that occurs with exercise. The choices of protein are based on how the body will break them down. First-choice protein sources include lean meats, such as fat-trimmed beef or pork, chicken, white tuna in water, and nonfried seafood. Second choice sources will come from dairy, nuts, and seeds, and include milk, soy milk, yogurt, beans, peas, lentils, soy foods, and peanut butter.

## Fat

Fat is the secondary source of energy, and is often utilized during long bouts of exercise or activity. It is an essential part of the body's composition and must be included in the athlete's diet. Many diet and nutritional books advocate avoiding fats, but realize the body needs fats to protect the organs and maximize athletic composition. Of course, there are good fats and bad fats. *Saturated fat*, is the bad fat the body does not need, most often found in fried foods, fast foods, and in animal fats like cheese, cream, and butter. *Polyunsaturated fats* should be limited, and are found in vegetable oils and processed margarine. The best fats are *monounsaturated fats*, found in whole foods such as olives, extra-virgin olive oil, avocados, fish, clams, oysters, scallops, nuts, and natural peanut butter.

## CALORIC INTAKE

The essential thing to understand about caloric intake is the simple concept of input versus output. Calories are a way to measure the energy value of a food product. An athlete's caloric intake for the day is dictated by how much energy will be expended that day. A high-activity day requires higher consumption. Conversely, a low-activity day will not have as much caloric demand, and consumption should be lower.

If an athlete is programming for weight loss or gain, caloric intake may need to be further adjusted. Baseline caloric intake can be calculated by multiplying body weight in pounds times 15. For example, a 150-pound athlete must consume 2,250 calories per day in order to maintain his or her current body weight. Work from this baseline to accommodate for higher- and lower-activity days, and adjust the total caloric intake based on goals of weight gain or loss.

## SUPPLEMENT AND STEROID ABUSE IN THE SOCCER PLAYER

Everything an athlete can gain from supplementation can be achieved through proper nutrition. However, a busy, active lifestyle can make it difficult to always eat a proper meal. Subsequently, athletes may have a hard time obtaining all the proper daily nutrients from food choices alone, and will look to supplementation to bridge this gap in their diets. It is always wise to consult a physician who knows your medical background and can make an educated recommendation about supplementation before deciding on a product to use. Keep in mind that the FDA does not regulate the dietary supplement industry, which means it is impossible to truly know what you are putting into your body. This is especially important if competing in the National Collegiate Athletic Association (NCAA), as there may be a banned substance in the manufacturer's "proprietary blend" that can cause a failed drug test. Even more importantly, if you don't know what you're putting into your body, you may be putting yourself at a major health risk.

No human being should be adding anything into his or her diet if they don't know exactly what it is, especially if the decision is not guided by a physician or nutritionist. Too many times, decisions are made by looking in the mirror, and not by getting the appropriate urinalysis to see if the body is indeed lacking any nutrients. It's my opinion that you should not put any man-made supplements into your body unless approved after testing. Research shows that 65% to 75% of added vitamins and minerals cannot be properly absorbed and literally end up in the toilet bowl; basically you're flushing your money down the toilet.

Many athletes want to use some sort of protein or creatine supplement to add muscle mass and aid in muscle recovery. These products can safely be used for exactly those reasons, but it is important for the athlete to understand that more is not always better, especially because supplement abuse can sometimes lead to steroid abuse.

## HARMFUL EFFECTS OF SUPPLEMENTATION AND STEROID ABUSE

Think of the body as a storage room with shelves. If looking at the different nutrients on each labeled shelf, the body, through foods and a multivitamin, will fill each shelf accordingly. When the shelves are full, the body cannot absorb any more, and will need to work harder to flush out the excess. Oversupplementation can overstress the digestive system, liver, stomach, and pancreas and can potentially result in damage to the system.

A more immediate threat comes from products acting as "accelerants." These products claim to help the body get lean or more "cut." Common sense says if you're taking something to speed up metabolism, and your heart rate along with it, your heart will eventually get tired and fail. Why would anyone, especially an athlete, want to speed up their heart prior to exercise? This is a major risk for any athlete, and should never be a part of anyone's diet.

Unfortunately, some soccer athletes will skip over the supplement stage and jump directly into steroid use. It is important to understand that steroids are drugs. They are man-made substances related to the male sex hormone testosterone. Medically, some are used for various pathologies and can be used for good, but when abused by athletes, steroids always cause more harm than good.

People use the big words "anabolic," or muscle-building, and "androgenic," which refers to masculine characteristics, when describing steroids. Athletes are always looking for an edge, and steroids will give you that edge. You will get bigger, faster, and stronger, but not without harmful, unavoidable side effects.

**Side Effects of Steroids in Males**

- Shrinking of testicles
- Infertility
- Baldness
- Increased breast size
- Increased risk of cancer

**Side Effects of Steroids in Females**

- Changes to your menstrual cycle
- Deepened voice
- Male characteristics, such as facial hair or male pattern baldness
- Long-term effects from depleted estrogen
- Infertility
- Increased risk of cancer

Other harmful effects of steroids in children and young athletes are accelerated puberty, premature growth and shortening of growth plates, liver tumors, fluid retention, increase in low-density lipoprotein or bad cholesterol, decrease in high-density lipoprotein or good cholesterol, kidney tumors, severe acne, and tremors. If steroids are injected, HIV and AIDS are also risks. Steroids can also have psychological effects, such as aggression, mood swings, and invincibility traits.

I understand that soccer athletes face pressures from a variety of sources. Parents, coaches, peers, and teammates expect the athlete to perform. The athlete wants to get a scholarship or financial aid or go pro, and he or she may view supplements and steroids as a shortcut to success. But steroids are drugs and they are illegal, and using them at any level is cheating. If an athlete feels he or she needs an additional edge, there are nutrition professionals available for consultation. They're all able to help athletes achieve their nutritional goals and maximize their athletic potential. But remember, nothing can replace hard work!

# JAG PHYSICAL THERAPY LESS PROGRAM

My LESS program is designed to strengthen the lower body for athletes to provide a better base of support during athletic activity, or everyday life. The lower body is the base of our structure, so keeping it strong during physical activity is extremely important. Strengthening the lower body assists in prevention of common injuries such as ACL, MCL, LCL, and PCL tears and sprains, meniscus tears, hip labral tears, hip flexor strains, groin pulls, ankle sprains, calf strains, shin splints, and stress fractures.

The program is three days a week to allow for appropriate rest and recovery in between sessions. The program is three weeks long and each week builds upon the next. When the program has been completed, the third week of exercises should be incorporated into a regular training program, continued at least two to three times a week.

| JAG PHYSICAL THERAPY LOWER EXTREMITY STRENGTHENING SYSTEM | | | |
|---|---|---|---|
| | **WEEK 2**<br>**DAY 1** | **WEEK 2**<br>**DAY 2** | **WEEK 2**<br>**DAY 3** |
| **Warm-Up** | • Forward jogging (2 min)<br>• Shuttle (switch midway) (2 min)<br>• Backward jogging (2 min)<br>• Hip swings (all planes, 30 s)<br>• 50% quick feet (50 ft forward/backward)<br>• Progressive skipping →High skips →Bounding (50 ft each)<br>• Long stride backward (50 ft) | • Forward jogging (2 min)<br>• Shuttle (switch midway) (2 min)<br>• Backward jogging (2 min)<br>• Hip swings (all planes, 30 s)<br>• 50% quick feet (50 ft forward/backward)<br>• Progressive skipping → High skips → Bounding (50 ft each)<br>• Long stride backward (50 ft) | • Forward jogging (2 min)<br>• Shuttle (switch midway) (2 min)<br>• Backward jogging (2 min)<br>• Hip swings (all planes, 30 s)<br>• 50% quick feet (50 ft forward/backward)<br>• Progressive skipping → High skips → Bounding (50 ft each)<br>• Long stride backward (50 ft) |
| **Stretching** | • Supine hamstring stretch (with strap)<br>• Figure 4 Stretch (piriformis, Figure 2.4)<br>• Abductor and adductor stretch (with strap)<br>• Side lying quad stretch (opposite knee bent)<br>• Pyramid calf stretches (knee straight and bent) | • Supine hamstring stretch (with strap)<br>• Figure 4 Stretch (piriformis)<br>• Abductor and adductor stretch (with strap)<br>• Side lying quad stretch (opposite knee bent)<br>• Pyramid calf stretches (knee straight and bent) | • Supine hamstring stretch (with strap)<br>• Figure 4 Stretch (piriformis)<br>• Abductor and adductor stretch (with strap)<br>• Side lying quad stretch (opposite knee bent)<br>• Pyramid calf stretches (knee straight and bent) |

| Jumping | • 2 leg broad jump<br>• 2 leg box jumps<br>• 2 Leg 90° squat jump<br>• 2 leg side hurdle jump<br>• 2 leg 180° jumps | • 2 leg 90° squat jump<br>• 2 leg side hurdle jump<br>• 2 leg hurdle jump (stick landing)<br>• 1 leg hop (forward/backward)<br>• 2 leg box jumps<br>• 2 leg 180° jumps | • 2 leg 90° squat jump<br>• 2 leg side hurdle jump (stick landing)<br>• 1 leg hurdle jump (stick landing)<br>• 1 leg hop (forward/backward)<br>• 1 leg side hurdle hops<br>• 2 leg 180° jumps |
|---|---|---|---|
| **Strengthening** | • Bridges on ball (10x, 3 s hold) (Figure 8)<br>• Single leg bridge on ball (10x, 3 s hold) (Figure 9)<br>• Romanian dead lift (bent knee) (10x)<br>• Walking lunge (10x)<br>• Quadruped superman (alternate arm/leg) (Figure 10) | • Bridges on ball (10x, 3 s hold)<br>• Single leg bridge on ball (10x, 3 s hold)<br>• Romanian dead lift (bent knee) (10x)<br>• Walking lunge (10x)<br>• Quadruped superman (alternate arm/leg) | • Bridges on ball (10x, 3 s hold)<br>• Single leg bridge on ball (10x, 3 s hold)<br>• Romanian dead lift (bent knee) (10x)<br>• Walking lunge (10x)<br>• Quadruped superman (alternate arm/leg) |

## JAG PHYSICAL THERAPY LOWER EXTREMITY STRENGTHENING SYSTEM

| | WEEK 1 DAY 1 | WEEK 1 DAY 2 | WEEK 1 DAY 3 |
|---|---|---|---|
| **Warm-Up** | • Forward jogging (2 min)<br>• Shuttle (switch midway) (2 min)<br>• Backward jogging (2 min)<br>• Hip swings (all planes, 30 s)<br>• 50% quick feet (50 ft forward/backward)<br>• Progressive skipping →High skips→Bounding (50 ft each)<br>• Long stride backward (50 ft) | • Forward jogging (2 min)<br>• Shuttle (switch midway) (2 min)<br>• Backward jogging (2 min)<br>• Hip swings (all planes, 30 s)<br>• 50% quick feet (50 ft forward/backward)<br>• Progressive skipping →High skips →Bounding (50 ft each)<br>• Long stride backward (50 ft) | • Forward jogging (2 min)<br>• Shuttle (switch midway) (2 min)<br>• Backward jogging (2 min)<br>• Hip swings (all planes, 30 s)<br>• 50% quick feet (50 ft forward/backward)<br>• Progressive skipping →High skips →Bounding (50 ft each)<br>• Long stride backward (50 ft) |
| **Stretching** | • Supine hamstring stretch (with strap) (Figure 6.10)<br>• Figure 4 Stretch (piriformis, Figure 2.4)<br>• Abductor and adductor stretch (with strap) (Figures 1 and 2)<br>• Side lying quad stretch (opposite knee bent) (Figure 3)<br>• Pyramid calf stretches (knee straight and bent) (Figure 4) | • Supine hamstring stretch (with strap)<br>• Figure 4 Stretch (piriformis)<br>• Abductor and adductor stretch (with strap)<br>• Side lying quad stretch (opposite knee bent)<br>• Pyramid calf stretches (knee straight and bent) | • Supine hamstring stretch (with strap)<br>• Figure 4 Stretch (piriformis)<br>• Abductor and adductor stretch (with strap)<br>• Side lying quad stretch (opposite knee bent)<br>• Pyramid calf stretches (knee straight and bent) |

| | | | |
|---|---|---|---|
| **Jumping** | <ul><li>2 leg vertical jumps (10x, 45 s recovery)</li><li>Squat jumps</li><li>2 leg box jumps</li><li>2 leg side jumps</li><li>2 leg forward</li><li>2 leg backward jumps</li><li>2 leg 90° jump</li></ul> | <ul><li>2 leg vertical jumps (10x, 45 s recovery)</li><li>Squat jumps</li><li>2 leg box jumps</li><li>2 leg side jumps</li><li>2 leg forward</li><li>2 leg backward jumps</li><li>2 leg 90° jump</li></ul> | <ul><li>2 leg vertical jumps (10x, 45 s recovery)</li><li>Squat jumps</li><li>2 leg box jumps</li><li>2 leg side box jumps (if proper form)</li><li>2 leg forward</li><li>2 leg backward jumps</li><li>2 leg 90° jump</li></ul> |
| **Strengthening** | <ul><li>Bridges (10x, 3 s hold) (Figure 5)</li><li>Single leg bridge (10x, 3 s hold) (Figure 6)</li><li>Romanian dead lift (bent knee) (10x)</li><li>Walking lunge (10x)</li><li>Prone supermans (10x) (Figure 7)</li><li>Planks (30 s)</li></ul> | <ul><li>Bridges (10x, 3 s hold)</li><li>Single leg bridge (10x, 3 s hold)</li><li>Romanian dead lift (bent knee) (10x)</li><li>Walking lunge (10x)</li><li>Prone supermans (10x)</li><li>Planks (30 s)</li></ul> | <ul><li>Bridges (10x, 3 s hold)</li><li>Single leg bridge (10x, 3 s hold)</li><li>Romanian dead lift (bent knee) (10x)</li><li>Walking lunge (10x)</li><li>Prone supermans (10x)</li><li>Planks (30 s)</li></ul> |

| JAG PHYSICAL THERAPY LOWER EXTREMITY STRENGTHENING SYSTEM | | | |
|---|---|---|---|
| | **WEEK 3 DAY 1** | **WEEK 3 DAY 2** | **WEEK 3 DAY 3** |
| **Warm-Up** | • Forward jogging (2 min)<br>• Shuttle (switch midway) (2 min)<br>• Backward jogging (2 min)<br>• Hip swings (all planes, 30 s)<br>• 50% quick feet (50 ft forward/backward)<br>• Progressive skipping → High skips → Bounding (50 ft each)<br>• Long stride backward (50 ft) | • Forward jogging (2 min)<br>• Shuttle (switch midway) (2 min)<br>• Backward jogging (2 min)<br>• Hip swings (all planes, 30 s)<br>• 50% quick feet (50 ft forward/backward)<br>• Progressive skipping → High skips → Bounding (50 ft each)<br>• Long stride backward (50 ft) | • Forward jogging (2 min)<br>• Shuttle (switch midway) (2 min)<br>• Backward jogging (2 min)<br>• Hip swings (all planes, 30 s)<br>• 50% quick feet (50 ft forward/backward)<br>• Progressive skipping → High skips → Bounding (50 ft each)<br>• Long stride backward (50 ft) |
| **Stretching** | • Supine hamstring stretch (with strap)<br>• Figure 4 Stretch (piriformis, Figure 2.4)<br>• Abductor and adductor stretch (with strap)<br>• Side lying quad stretch (opposite knee bent)<br>• Pyramid calf stretches (knee straight and bent) | • Supine hamstring stretch (with strap)<br>• Figure 4 Stretch (piriformis)<br>• Abductor and adductor stretch (with strap)<br>• Side lying quad stretch (opposite knee bent)<br>• Pyramid calf stretches (knee straight and bent) | • Supine hamstring stretch (with strap)<br>• Figure 4 Stretch (piriformis)<br>• Abductor and adductor stretch (with strap)<br>• Side lying quad Stretch (opposite knee bent)<br>• Pyramid calf stretches (knee straight and bent) |

| | | | |
|---|---|---|---|
| **Jumping** | • 2 leg hurdle jumps (with bounce)<br>• 1 leg hurdle jumps (with bounce)<br>• 1 leg forward/backward hops (with bounce)<br>• Ice skater forward (stick landing) (Figure 11)<br>• Ice skater backward (stick landing) (Figure 12)<br>• 2 leg 270° jumps | • 2 leg hurdle jumps (with bounce)<br>• 1 leg hurdle jumps (with bounce)<br>• 1 leg forward/backward hops (with bounce)<br>• Ice skater forward (stick landing)<br>• Ice skater backward (stick landing)<br>• 2 leg 270° jumps | • 2 leg hurdle jumps (with bounce)<br>• 1 leg hurdle jumps (with bounce)<br>• 1 leg forward/backward hops (with bounce)<br>• Ice skater forward (stick landing)<br>• Ice skater backward (stick landing)<br>• 2 leg 270° jumps |
| **Strengthening** | • Roll-in bridge on ball (10x, 3 s hold)<br>• Single leg bridge on ball (10x, 3 s hold)<br>• Single leg romanian dead lift (bent knee) (10x)<br>• Walking lunge (10x)<br>• Lunge series (10x)<br>• Hip band walking (lateral and monster) (Figure 13 and 14)<br>• Quadruped superman | • Roll-in bridge on ball (10x, 3 s hold)<br>• Single leg bridge on ball (10x, 3 s hold)<br>• Single leg romanian dead lift (bent knee) (10x)<br>• Walking lunge (10x)<br>• Lunge series (10x)<br>• Hip band walking (lateral and monster)<br>• Quadruped superman | • Roll-in bridge on ball (10x, 3 s hold)<br>• Single leg bridge on ball (10x, 3 s hold)<br>• Single leg romanian dead lift (bent knee) (10x)<br>• Walking lunge (10x)<br>• Lunge series (10x)<br>• Hip band walking (lateral and monster)<br>• Quadruped superman |

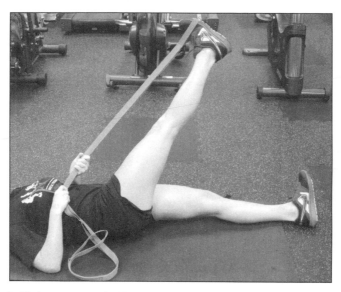

**Figure 1** Abductor stretch: Keeping your knee straight, pull your leg up off the ground and across the midline of your body. You should mostly feel this on the outside of your thigh, in your abductors.

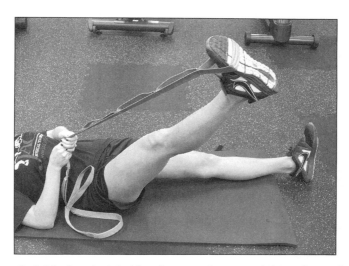

**Figure 2** Adductor stretch: Keeping your knee straight, pull your leg up off the ground and away from your body. You should mostly feel this on the inside of your thigh, in your adductors.

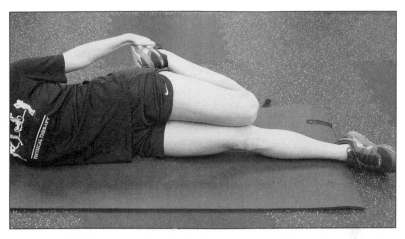

**Figure 3** Side lying quad stretch: Lying on your side, pull your foot up toward your buttock for a good quadriceps stretch.

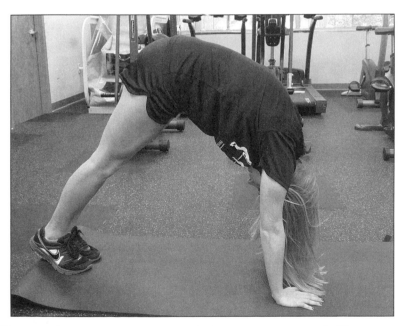

**Figure 4** Pyramid calf stretch: Begin lying on your stomach. Elevate your hips toward the sky, and with straight arms and legs, walk your hands back toward your feet to stretch out your calves.

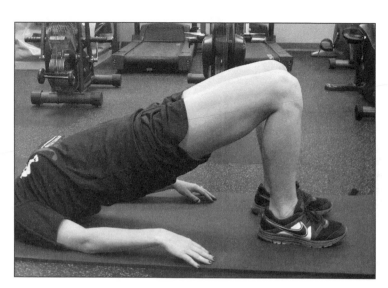

**Figure 5** Bridges: Keeping your feet firmly planted on the ground, elevate your hips up toward the sky, and maintain a straight line with your shoulder, hip, and knee. This activates your core musculature, mainly your glutes and hamstrings.

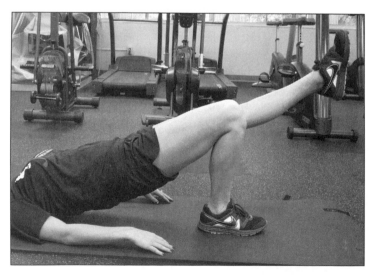

**Figure 6** Single leg bridge: Keeping one foot firmly planted on the ground with your other knee extended out, elevate your hips up toward the sky, and maintain a straight line with your shoulder, hip, and knee. This is a more advanced core exercise, adding an increased strength and stability component.

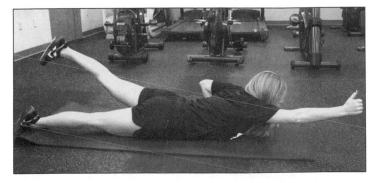

**Figure 7** Prone supermans: Lying on your stomach, elevate opposite arms and legs to activate your posterior core musculature.

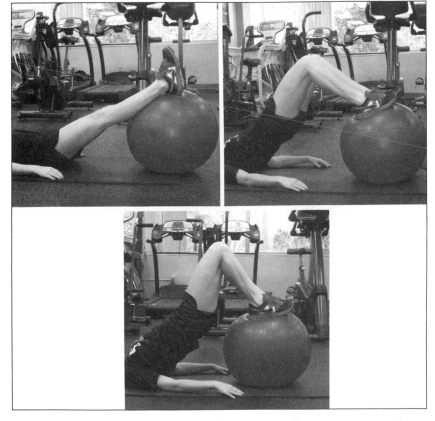

**Figure 8** Bridge on ball and roll-in bridge on ball: This is an advanced version of the table bridge. The ball adds a crucial stability component that challenges your core musculature. Begin in the first position at top left with your back flat on the floor. Pull your heels back toward your buttock, as in the top right image above. To do a roll-in bridge on ball, pull your heels in further, as in the image at bottom center.

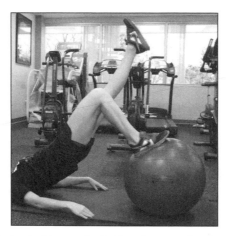

**Figure 9** Single leg bridge on ball: Keeping one foot in contact with the ball, with your other knee extended out, elevate your hips up toward the sky, and maintain a straight line with your shoulder, hip, and knee. This further advances the single leg bridge exercise, increasing stability and strength demands.

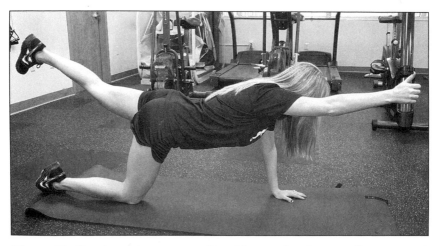

**Figure 10** Quadruped superman: On all fours, elevate opposite arms and legs to activate your posterior core musculature. Ideally, your hips will stay square to the floor with minimal rotation.

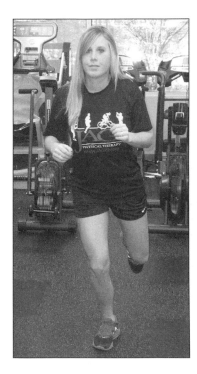

**Figure 11** Ice skater forward: Perform a short jump forward, while landing on a single leg. The idea is to maintain good positioning with your knees behind your toes and hips externally rotated.

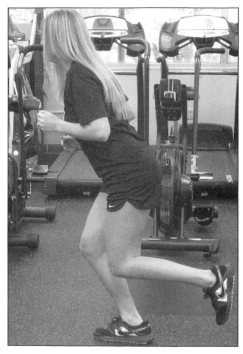

**Figure 12** Ice skater backward: Perform a short jump backward (90° rotation), while landing on a single leg. The idea is to maintain good positioning with your knees behind your toes and hips externally rotated.

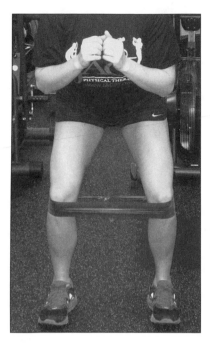

**Figure 13** Hip band walking lateral: Keeping a firm base and tight core, perform a lateral walk, side-stepping to the side. The idea is to maintain this position with your knees in good position behind your toes and external rotation at the hips (pushing them apart against the band).

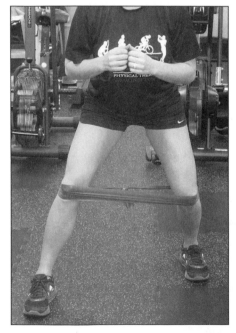

**Figure 14** Hip band walking monster: Similar to the lateral walk, maintain a firm base and tight core while taking short steps forward. Ideally, keep your feet wide while activating your hip abductors.

# GLOSSARY

**Ambulation**   Walking under an individual's own power, without assistance.

**Atrophy**   A muscular effect whereby mass is lost due to inactivity, commonly seen in the postinjured athlete.

**Avulsion**   A fracture that often occurs from a strong ligamentous pull that, rather than damaging the ligament, actually pulls the ligament away from its bony insertion, with the bone fragment still intact.

**Bilateral**   A directional term indicating both the right and left sides of the body.

**Bursa**   Fluid-filled sacs that act as lubricants in joint motion between tendon and bone.

**Bursitis**   An inflammatory response of the bursa sac, caused by either friction or direct impact.

**Closed kinetic chain exercise**   A form of exercise in which a limb is in contact with either the ground or another stable surface, such as a wall or table. The kinetic chain is activated with the foot or hand in contact with a surface and alters the effect of muscular action mostly by way of co-contraction.

**Co-contraction**   The action of opposing muscles against one another that helps to stabilize a joint throughout its range of motion.

**Commotio cordis**   A sudden cardiac arrest caused by a direct blow to the chest.

**Contralateral**   A directional term denoting the side of the body opposite that on which a particular injury or condition occurs; if talking about the right arm, the contralateral side is the left side.

**Dermatome**   An area of skin innervated by sensory fibers from a single spinal nerve.

**Distal**   A directional term indicating the farthest point away from the center of the body, or away from a point of attachment.

**Dorsiflexion**   Ankle motion in which the foot is flexed upward toward the shin. For example, toes to nose.

**Edema**   Swelling of tissue due to the body's inflammatory process.

**Erythema**   Redness of the skin caused by injury or infection.

**Eversion**   Ankle motion deriving from the subtalar joint, where the foot is extended away from the midline of the body, in an outward direction.

**Extensibility**   A muscle or tendon's ability to be stretched.

**Frontal plane**   A vertical plane that divides the body into front and back sections. Also known as the coronal plane.

**Functional exercise**   An exercise that incorporates the entire body in preparation for the activities of daily life, like squatting down and lifting an object.

**Hypertrophy**   An increase in muscle mass or girth through exercise.

**Hypertrophic cardiomyopathy**   A sometimes fatal condition in which a thickening of the heart muscle creates an inefficiency in the pumping of blood to the body.

**Inferior**   A directional term indicating below or underneath, or referring to the lower part of a structure or the lower of two similar structures.

**Inflammatory response**   The body's natural response to injury or infection, in which blood flow is stimulated to an area to "clean out" damaged tissue and replace with new tissue.

**Inversion**   Ankle motion deriving from the subtalar joint, in which the foot is extended inward toward the midline of the body.

**Ipsilateral**   A directional term indicating the same side of the body; if talking about the right arm, the ipsilateral side is the right side.

**Jone's fracture**   A fracture at the base of the fifth metatarsal bone in the foot.

**Labrum**   A ring of cartilage surrounding the socket portion of both the hip and shoulder joints that acts as a smooth point of contact for motion and helps maintain the stability of the joint.

**Lateral**   A directional term indicating an area away from the midline of the body; to the side.

**Lisfranc injury**   A fracture to the bones or injury to the ligaments of the Lisfranc joint, which consists of the five bones that make up the arch in the mid-foot.

**Medial**   A directional term indicating an area toward the midline of the body.

**Mechanism of injury (MOI)**   The manner in which various body tissues absorb stress and are subsequently damaged. MOI is a strong indicator of what structures are likely damaged and is an important piece of information for accurate evaluation of an injury.

**Mortise**   The joint space at the ankle, made up of the talus, distal tibia, and fibula bones.

**Mild traumatic brain injury (MTBI)**   A loss or alteration of consciousness caused by either a single impact to the head or multiple subconcussive impacts over time.

**Muscle guarding**   An immediate muscular response to an injury in which an involuntary muscular contraction acts to protect the injured limb.

**Muscle inhibition**   The inability of a muscle to contract in the days following injury, caused by a loss of neuromuscular control.

**Muscle setting exercise**   A therapeutic exercise used to restore neuromuscular control to an injured limb, such as quad sets.

**Open kinetic chain exercise**   A form of exercise in which no limbs are in contact with a stable surface, such as the ground or a wall or table. The kinetic chain is activated in an open-ended manner and alters the effect of muscular action on a joint by decreasing joint compressive forces and eliminating co-contraction.

**Pes cavus**  A foot shape with a pronounced arch and increased supination—a high instep.

**Pes planus**  A foot shape with essentially no arch, with the medial foot in contact with the ground—flat-footed.

**Plantarflexion**  Ankle motion in which the toes are pointed downward toward the ground.

**Platelet-rich plasma (PRP) injection**  A method of therapy in which an individual's own blood is spun in a centrifuge to remove the dense plasma, which is then injected directly into the site of musculoskeletal injury to promote healing.

**Progressive resistive exercises (PRE)**  An exercise plan in which a foundation is formed prior to increasing weights or resistance.

**Prone**  A body position in which an individual lies face down on the floor or table.

**Proprioception**  The body's awareness of a joint's or limb's relative position in time and space. Proprioceptive exercises, done with the eyes closed, help to increase this awareness.

**Proximal**  A directional term indicating the closest point toward the center of the body, or closer to a point of attachment.

**Range of motion**  The distance a joint can move between the flexed position and the extended position.

**Retinaculum**  Thin, fibrous bands of connective tissue that encapsulate groups of tendons around the joints and hold them in place.

**Sagittal plane**  The vertical plane that passes from front to back, dividing the body into right and left halves.

**Sport-specific exercise**  Any exercise designed to mimic the demands of a particular sport or position.

**Sprain**  A ligamentous injury, often resulting from an overstretching of the tissue, ranging in severity from grades 1 to 3.

**Strain**  A musculotendinous injury, often resulting from an overstretching of the tissue, ranging in severity from grades 1 to 3.

**Superior**  A directional term indicating above or on top of, or toward the head.

**Supine**   A body position in which an individual is lying flat on the floor or a table with the face up.

**Syndesmosis**   An articulation, allowing for a minimal range of motion, in which two bones are connected.

**Tendinitis**   An inflammatory response within a tendon or tendon sheath resulting in pain and loss of function.

**Transverse plane**   A horizontal plane that divides the body in half from top to bottom, perpendicular to the sagittal and frontal planes.

**Valgus stress**   Stress applied to any joint that is directed in a lateral to medial manner and creates a stretching of tissue on the medial (inside) aspect of the joint.

**Varus stress**   Stress applied to any joint that is directed in a medial to lateral manner and creates a stretching of tissue on the lateral (outside) aspect of the joint.

# ACKNOWLEDGMENTS

I would like to thank Kayla Devlin for her support, organizational skills, patience, and work ethic in assisting with this project each and every day. You assisted in making a dream come true.

I give my sincere thank you to David Motisi for his tireless hours upon hours in assisting to get the words out of my head and onto paper. You the man!

I want to extend a huge thank you to Lindsay Berra for her great work. Your writing and editing skills made this book something very special and a pleasure to read. I could not have done this without your efforts.

Joseph Persico, Erin Quinn, and Kayla Devlin, thank you for your assistance in demonstrating proper body mechanics for our illustrations. It will assist in decreasing numerous injuries.

Thank you to the entire JAG Physical Therapy staff for their support throughout the entirety of this project. Go Team JAG!!!

# INDEX

# ABOUT THE AUTHOR

John Gallucci, Jr., MS, ATC, PT, DPT, is the medical coordinator for Major League Soccer (MLS), overseeing the medical care of more than 600 professional soccer players, and the president of JAG Physical Therapy, managing eight outpatient, physical therapy sports medicine centers in New York and New Jersey. Gallucci serves as a medical resource to over 100 soccer clubs throughout New York and New Jersey for athletic training services, injury prevention education, and the highest quality sports-medicine physical therapy care as well as a sports medicine consultant for many NFL, NHL, NBA, MLB, and MLS athletes. He has appeared on ESPN's award-winning *Outside the Lines*, Fox 5 News, and WFAN, and has been featured in New York's *Daily News* and *First for Women*, among numerous other media outlets.

www.jagpt.com